ABC of CARE

A handbook for home caregivers

Madeleine Forell Marshall
© 2015

Neuromuscular disease is especially public and ghastly as a catastrophic disorder. So we have the ALS challenge and the inspirational movie about Stephen Hawking. But it's not uniquely awful and I often thought, during our ordeal and afterward that caring for a loved one with dementia or uncontrollable diabetes or inoperable cancer would be no less awful. Caring for a baby or any child would be a nightmare of fear and hope, pity and love, sleeplessness and despair.

I am a Christian and my husband was a Lutheran pastor. For those who knew us this was a dimension of our six years of disability and care. But I have tried to put those realities in the background so as not to complicate the reading of my little primer. The book is for anybody who is faced with the realities and the choices, the burdens and the joys of caring—at home and in the hospital, in rehab and on the road—for another human being. It is also meant to help medical professionals, counselors and church people understand what's going on in the minds and hearts of patients and their families.

The format, the division of this book into short little segments is to honor the fragmented and interrupted life we live as caregivers. Alarms and phone calls, meals and medications, toileting and visits, stopping to shower or grab a sandwich—these shatter every day into many fragments. Snippets of experience, of lessons learned, these seemed best.

A

Advice

It was like being thrown into deep, deep, cold water without ever having learned to swim. After six months of creeping disability, my strong, capable husband had had surgery and now he couldn't walk. The hospital passed him along to a rehab facility. When he "failed" to rehabilitate, the rehab facility decided to send him home.

Home was upstairs and stairs were no longer possible. Nor could he negotiate the cramped spaces of our apartment in a wheelchair. The physical therapists who did a "home evaluation" confirmed the impossibility. The rehab hospital, working through their chain of advisers, found a "board and care" where I could stay with Gary and learn to care for him, or get my bearings, or at least learn to float!

At this point we had been advised to prepare for the end by one doctor who believed Gary had ALS and had watched a favorite mentor die of that disease. He described end stage ALS in grim terms, the lungs filling with fluid and the victim dying. The next visit the doctor shared his latest personal news—about having just bought a Porsche for his girlfriend. That was the last time I allowed him into our new and fragile sphere.

Within a few short months Gary would be unable to breathe or speak or eat on his own. Family and friends were devastated. He was a monument of strength and will and good grace.

I couldn't swim!

The world is full of advice for the new caregiver—of a child or a spouse or a parent or a friend. Officious advice from the people in the hospital paid to "manage" your care. Social workers and case managers and discharge nurses all know everything—or so they would have you believe. Various doctors and nurses, all doubtless well-intentioned, have stories to tell and ideas to share and theories and counsel. Some of it is excellent. Some is worthless. Some is dangerous.

One size does not fit all. Care may be for a week or a month or six months or a year or many years.

I was advised that home care was unreasonable. It would never work to care for somebody so disabled at home. Like so much advice, this seemed ridiculous, wrong, a terrible idea. I would learn. I would find a way. I would make this work. After almost six years, I can speak with some authority.

- Caveat: Key discharge staff are in cahoots with insurance companies and medical suppliers. They will load you up with all the medical equipment they can justify with insurance, including worthless items you will never use—commodes for people who cannot get out of bed, wheelchairs with fancy controls for people who can no longer move their hands, ridiculous, ugly old beds, and lots of those miserable, tacky bed socks. They will not supply you with bed pads, exam gloves, a blood pressure cuff or a hundred other supplies that are basic requirements for home care.

- Caveat: Dozens of people prey on the newly disabled and their care providers—transport specialists, nursing agencies, suppliers of oxygen and costly infusion therapies, insurance company "patient advocates" and always, social workers. We never needed oxygen tanks. They rolled around in the garage for years. According to one company, they could only be removed from our home with a doctor's prescription. Meanwhile, the oxygen company, the only source of advice here, raked in the profits.

You cannot know what you do not need. You cannot know which advice is sound and which is really dumb. You cannot trust anybody and have to trust everybody.

- Caveat: Beware of rehabilitation. Three years into our ordeal, my father was visiting us when he fell and broke his hip. After the replacement surgery he was transferred to a rehab hospital where he slowly began to waste away. He was almost ninety and the staff did what was required and then left him with no batteries in his hearing aids, no stimulation, sharing a depressing room with another hopeless case. Practiced (lamentably) in the ways of insurance, I enlisted a friendly doctor, procured a portable oxygen concentrator, essentially kidnapped my father from rehab and packed him on a plane home. The rehab hospital wasn't going to let him go until all his Medicare rehab days were used up, even if that meant leaving in a hearse. (My father lived another two years, thank you, and died peacefully at home.)

Amateurs

This is very much the book of an amateur, written for other amateurs. Professionals are trained; they are taught. In nursing programs the instruction begins with very basic science and very basic skills and slowly, over the months, new understanding of the theory and practice of nursing are built up. Amateurs, like me, are another story. We are suddenly, with no desire and no preparation, expected to do all kinds of crazy things. And to do them when we are frightened and exhausted, depressed and aghast.

I had to learn all sorts of skills that were simply unimaginable to me before our "fall" into disability. Every two days I emptied my husband's bowels with my gloved fingers. Every two weeks I supervised the replacement of his "suprapubic catheter," the tube that went through his abdominal wall into his bladder. I fed him through another tube, crushed pills and pushed them into his stomach. The list was very long. I could (and did) replace the whole apparatus that delivered air through his throat into his lungs, a terrifying project as every second mattered and there was no margin for error.

Most remarkably, I became practiced in transferring him from his bed, in loading the huge wheelchair into the van, in troubleshooting equipment failures and talking other people through one or another scary situation, often over the phone. As an amateur, I had to correct all sorts of professionals who were messing up.

We tend to think there are experts to whom to turn. Not so. Many of the experts are ignorant or unimaginative. I have been told ridiculous things, given ridiculous instructions. All too often amateurs are discredited rather than empowered. This little primer is designed to counteract the denigration of amateurs.

B

Beasy Boards, Lifts and the Silent Knight

Perhaps I have been hard on the discharge planners and the load of insurance-approved supplies they order up for your home. These supplies are called **Durable Medical Equipment** or "DME" in the parlance of home care. (See Wikipedia.) That's the technical term for what I came long ago to think of as "handicrap"—commode (i.e. adult potty) chairs, shiny "Hoyer" lifts, transfer boards and wheelchairs, hospital beds and breathing machines. Each has a use. It may not suit your purposes or practices but you won't know that until you've tried.

Transfer boards are simple, varnished wooden boards that may well work for her strapping son or daughter to shift a weak little old lady from bed to wheelchair. Physical therapists impressively use them for larger patients, often in conjunction with a "gait belt." Do not try this yourself! They are ridiculously inadequate for a normal person moving a normal-size or large patient from bed to chair. You'll kill your back and drop your beloved husband or wife, life partner or good friend on the floor.

One clever solution is a "Beasy Board," available online. A plastic disc slides along a track in a plastic arc and, deployed just so, glides the patient from bed (at the right height or a bit above) to chair (arm lowered) with something like ease. Insurance does not pay for Beasy Boards but does pay for your back therapy. (No, this is not reasonable.)

The hospital may send you home with a mechanical (hydraulic) "Hoyer lift" and a sling. You roll your patient onto the sling, position the lift legs under the bed, attach the sling loops to the lift hooks and pump the handle until your loved one is hanging in midair. This lets you move him or her over the wheelchair. You then release the hydraulics and lower your patient into the chair. Manual Hoyer lifts are to nicely engineered electric lifts as transfer boards are to the Beasy variety.

My Norwegian-engineered Molift collapsed to fit in the trunk of a car. (It went with us to hotels.) It can position a patient in the right car—not my little compact. The wheels don't jam from collecting fibers and hair. The battery charge lasts for weeks. The whole system is so stable I could use it to haul my husband out to the living room, where he settled into his "zero gravity" recliner. And the grandchildren simply loved to play with the Molift, swinging from the sling and raising one another from the floor to midair and down again.

I maintained from day one that any pleasure or delight anyone could obtain from our medical catastrophe was the purest sort of joy. So the children made balloons from exam gloves, turned feeding syringes into water cannons and played dentist with the discarded nebulizer. The littlest babies slept cradled on their grandpa's chest, which rose and fell with each breath from the ventilator. So he listened on his headphones to the inane television shows chosen by his beloved granddaughter and the babies used his "chux" as changing pads.

Sometimes what you need hasn't been thought of yet and friends have to step in. Moving my husband to the living room used to require some second person staggering alongside the lift, hauling the heavy ventilator, ensuring that none of the tubes came loose. A simple piece of plywood, snapping onto the lift legs and carved to hold the vent solved the whole problem, thanks to Bob Foulke. A manual "tilt-in-space" wheelchair that I bought on eBay lacked a "vent tray." A clever caregiver fashioned a strong compartment out of metal strapping that worked better than the official vent tray on the fancy motorized chair. (Thanks, Joseph Rivera.)

Another crucial piece of equipment was devised for Gary by a chiropractor and designed to extend his lower back. It was basically a trapeze that suspended with two lengths of chain from the frame of the Molift. When I put the bar of the trapeze under Gary's knees and attached the chains to the Molift, I could raise his lower body off the bed. I sometimes swung him gently from side to side.

But the trapeze was most useful for moving Gary up in the bed. After three or four turns, he had always slipped down in the bed. When down in the bed the bend could curl his upper back and restrict his breathing. Unassisted, it was almost impossible for me to raise him up in the bed. But when, using the trapeze, I had lifted his lower body above the bed, then I was strong enough to raise his head to the top of the mattress and we were good for another three or four turns—or until help arrived.

Wheelchair sales, wheelchair repair, wheelchair science is a whole world unto itself. Our main wheelchair cost Aetna more than $26,000. It was a piece of junk. The physical therapist who worked for the manufacturer included all sorts of bells and whistles, like a "sip and puff" control but the chair didn't arrive until long after my husband lost that sort of control. The chair had many "drives" but jolted and jumped over a small seam in the sidewalk. It was supposed to be able to climb a one-inch curb but never could. In retrospect it was a fantasy purchase, letting us for a short while imagine the lives of the wheelchair hot rodders and other robustly disabled jocks who perform for the videos. It was never appropriate for us and it makes me crazy that we were saddled with such a machine.

I had to buy a van. Most of the taxis that claimed to haul people in wheelchairs couldn't accommodate my husband's huge chair. Those that could never came on time and we missed appointments. Getting to church was nearly impossible.

As with the wretched wheelchair, the only people with counsel on vans were the people selling the vehicles—not a good arrangement. They make a killing on the needs of the frantic, newly stricken disabled men and women and their families. So I went out and bought a van with serious adaptations—extended frame, electronic ramp, "kneeling" function that lowered the whole vehicle on the side my husband entered. As the chair was ordered for somebody who had a bit of control, so the van was really designed for somebody who could, by himself, trigger the ramp and enter the van. It was way more automation than we would need. We kept it. It worked. We traveled. But the system that had salespeople pushing an expensive product on clueless and stressed buyers is all wrong.

I shopped tirelessly on the internet for equipment, for timesavers, for laborsaving devices. These included many communication devices. There was the system that was supposed to track eye movements and allow my husband to move a cursor across the computer screen, selecting letters and typing. The software wasn't very stable however and using the system was very frustrating. I bought a bite switch which was supposed to allow him, using his teeth, to signal. That never worked very well either. Then there were the brainwave technologies—a couple of them. Hours and hours of placing and testing electrodes, hooking them up just so and trying to make sense of the results.

The Silent Knight was a long time coming. It's a pill crusher, required to crush pills so they can be dissolved in water and injected into a feeding tube. Hospitals and nursing homes use them. The pills are placed in a tough plastic pouch, then smashed to dust. Even big, fat vitamin tablets crumble in the Silent Knight. If pills aren't ground finely they jam in the feeding syringe or even the tube. This is a little crisis that can cause considerable aggravation, a wet mess in the bedclothes and loss of medication.

Before I bought a Silent Knight I tried half a dozen cheap plastic gizmos. None of them worked for more than a couple of weeks. The threads on the screws lost their grip. I tried hammering pills in plastic wrap, in baggies. I tried a rolling pin. I tried the coffee grinder. I bought a marble mortar and pestle at World Market. That worked fairly well—although pieces of pill would sometimes fly out—until somebody dropped the pestle and it cracked in pieces. Finally, in year four, I think it was, I bit the bullet and ordered up a Silent Knight. It worked well and saved stress. I'm only sorry I didn't spring for the thing early on.

Bodies and Boundaries

I suppose this entry is fundamentally about sex. One of the many challenges I have faced and that I suspect is faced by all husbands and wives of chronic patients is the jealousy of the body of the beloved. When some other woman is undressing or washing my husband, I am bothered.

We all begin life with basic teaching about modesty and privacy. From infancy, we are covered, protected, coached in discretion. This is culturally variable, of course, and some families are more modest than others. Some individuals are more unhappy about nudity than others. But the basic dilemma remains—that's my husband lying there, naked and exposed and vulnerable to your touch.

Certainly there are boundary issues here. My body has its boundaries. It stops here and yours begins there and you must have my permission to touch me and give me permission to touch you. Children who lack such boundaries are frequently victims of abuse. Women who lack such boundaries are often groped or molested. The healthy self bristles at unsolicited touch.

I believe that we are aware of similar boundaries containing those we love. So aggression directed at my beloved child is as awful as aggression directed at me. So another person bathing or cleaning, turning or massaging my husband provoked a strange sense of violation. It wasn't exactly jealousy but it may have been close.

After so many years, I learned to set this jealousy aside, but I remember well the affront in those early months. Having struggled to bathe and dress his inert body myself, relief at the help overcame the basic jealousy, but it remained real.

Sharing the care of a beloved body isn't precisely sexual, but there is, to be perfectly forthright, something strange going on. Those genitals that you are washing, those hands, those lips—they have given me much pleasure over many years and I love them more than you can possibly understand!

Business of Home Care

Managing home care of a chronic invalid is for all the world like managing a small business, something for which I was never trained. Sure, I have paid bills and organized files for the annual tax ordeal. I have comparison shopped and tried to make up and keep a budget. My husband and I had struggled over the years on a pastor's meager salary, paying off school debt and sometimes stressed over mortgage payments. We rarely had much extra and could certainly never afford long-term care insurance. We always assumed that the pension plan of the national church would cover our health and retirement needs.

While I can be bitter that was not so, I was more often grateful and even astonished that we managed to carry on financially.

Early in this journey, a relative of a friend who is an expert in "disability" advised me to "pay down" all of our assets so we would qualify for Medicaid. Medicaid payments were very generous for home care for somebody in my husband's condition. Upwards of $200,000 per year, the expert said. Our home could be sheltered but our other assets would have to go away. (This was before the crash of 2008, when Medicaid funding became shaky.)

The national church (ELCA) has a way to get rid of people who are severely disabled. First, they move you from their health insurance to Medicare as quickly as possible. Their health insurance pays for home nursing. In our case, that was 70 hours per week. The church advisors assured us that Medicare would cover as many as 35 hours per week—neglecting to explain that those hours were for charges like physical and occupational therapy sessions only available to patients on the mend. Those advisors were unrepentant and unremitting. Within eighteen months of my husband's disability, we were thrown on our own devices and I had to hustle to find resources to manage his care at home.

At any given time, I had from two to seven people on my "payroll." I had great nurses with questionable legal standing and at least one convicted felon working for me. I raided local nursing schools, hired heavily tattooed CNAs using Craigslist and found one truly demented caregiver (as well as several gems) on Care.com. I had numbers of nursing agencies offer to find help. They visited the house for lengthy "assessments," only to admit that their minimum hourly charge for help with my husband would cost close to $50.00 per hour. At $50 per hour we would indeed qualify for Medicaid in short order!

This was not a project I chose. This was not a business for which I had any identifiable qualifications. My only training in home care was a short unit in the Girl Scout Handbook, circa 1955, on the duties of a "Home Nurse."

I learned to use spreadsheets for recording medical expenses and payroll. I learned to manage multiple phone calls—while using my computer—on hold here, cut off there, working up the chain of customer service reps at medical supply companies. I learned to check insurance claims and argue patiently with clueless apparatchiks in call centers.

C

Caregiver Wellness

If you are a caregiver, dozens of people will tell you regularly to "take care of yourself." They will send you articles or cite alarming statistics about the bad health of caregivers who sacrifice their wellbeing and burn out or even drop dead from their exertions. The advisors most often seem to recommend "respite" or physically getting away from the loved person to whom you are devoted. Perhaps that's good advice, only perhaps. If everybody who advised respite or self-care would commit to learning the basics of spelling the caregiver—whatever the nursing demands—it would mean a lot more!

More urgent than getting away, it seems to me, are basic matters of diet and exercise. Whatever your age or level of fitness, you really need to figure out how to get stronger and healthier. This is hard, especially if you are panicked or depressed.

In the first stage of my husband's disability, self-care meant hauling the groceries upstairs and walking the dog. (That's basic strength training and moderate aerobic exercise.) A year later, after he was totally paralyzed, it meant hourly turns, using a draw sheet to roll his body from one side to the other, positioning pillows and raising the head of the bed. The laundry and the shopping, the hauling and the errands continued. (We had given the dog away.) That first year I lost a lot of weight. My appetite disappeared in the hospital although I was desperately thirsty all the time. I seem to remember that I lived on orange things—juice and Cheetos.

I gained the weight back and learned to salve the terrible stress of our situation with food. It was especially comforting to eat with friends and family and the amazing carryout in Los Angeles made for real pleasure. Think sushi and pizza, Chinese fusion and Cuban delicacies.

I had not fed myself ever. We had married young and I moved from college cafeteria fare to cooking for a hungry husband on a strict budget. Now we fed him cans of formula through his stomach tube and I was at a loss. I tried raw food. I tried living on fruit. I tried living on vegetables. I even tried cans and bars of Atkins this and South Beach that.

I went for walks in the park and even tried to jog—while paying caregivers $15 an hour to tend my man. I bought an elliptical trainer for home so I could exercise while "on duty" in the next room. It was dark and depressing.

Meanwhile, my doctor announced that my upper body fat was below 5%. The constant pushing and pulling and hauling my tall, heavy, inert husband meant that I was solid muscle through my back and shoulders.

I was very careful about my back. Early on, Gary joked about how my back was now our back. I had huge elastic braces that I wore at the first twinge of pain. I made the people I paid to help wear them as well and even thought about bringing them to the hospital to make the hospital nurses wear them! I stretched. I worked on the abs that support my "core." I bought large bottles of generic ibuprofen and handed them out like candy. I lay flat on the floor with my legs on the couch whenever I got the chance.

If I were to have had serious back trouble it would have been utterly catastrophic for our life together. If I couldn't have turned him every hour, my beloved husband would have had to go into a "facility," where he would have died within six weeks.

I like to imagine I could make a fortune writing a diet book, but every diet book I've ever read seems reducible to a simple list or two. The little lists are then hyped and expanded with feel-good, hopeful stories and pop science. Here's the essence of mine:

DIET:
1. Eat high-quality, low-fat protein at each meal:
    - Buy cartons of egg whites and cook with veggies or leftovers and grated cheese for breakfast.
    - Freeze individual packets of ham, fish, chicken breast, deli beef, shrimp, etc. They thaw in a flash and work for

- salads, sandwiches, or as an entrée with a mass of vegetables.
- Hard boil eggs for a quick snack, for egg salad, to add to green salad.
- Try "textured vegetable protein," which works as a high-protein oatmeal substitute (cooked in almond milk and served with slivered almonds and blueberries) or as a healthy version of ground beef (soaked in hot broth or even tomato soup).
- Don't overload on nuts, seeds and cheese, but they can save the hungry day.

2. Learn to eat vegetables rather than fruits. (This is a hard lesson because, obviously, fruits are sweet.)
    - Roast up a medley of vegetables tossed with olive oil at 435 for an hour. This will feed you for 3-4 days, including breakfast (sautéed with egg whites) and dinner (with or without a protein addition).
    - Keep raw vegetables in the fridge, prepared for snacking. Cream cheese or peanut butter complements these nicely.
    - Stir fry veggies with garlic and fresh ginger. Add half a can of cannellini beans, rinsed and drained, or garbanzos. Great with a glass of white wine.

3. Don't be mean to yourself, but know the perils of sweets, caffeine and alcohol.
    - If you have a sweet tooth, try sugar-free candy. (I find it hard to overindulge and tend to binge on anything else, including dried fruits.)
    - I find it comforting to bake cookies for church coffee hour, birthday cupcakes for the grandchildren, Christmas recipes for the holidays—all with the understanding that these aren't for ME.
    - I love coffee. I need coffee. I crave coffee. Good coffee, artisan roasted, with cream. I have, nevertheless, cut my fancy coffee with an equally good decaf, ordered from Amazon.com. This lets me drink coffee without tachycardia, a good thing. This compromise works for me.

- Alcohol: I can drink a whole bottle of wine by myself and I have done so. I can still perform all the emergency procedures my situation requires and I don't confuse the medications. I have never dropped my husband on the floor while inebriated or otherwise messed up. The next day I am neither hung over nor particularly unhappy. This is, however, not wise. Heavy drinking is not at all healthy. It does not make me a better person. It is expensive and probably dangerous.
- Therefore, I try to plan 3-4 "dry" days each week and to limit my alcohol to a glass or two on the other days. I drink champagne with family, celebrating new babies, life together, our general well-being. I suspect that alcohol and drugs are a major, unspoken factor in the lives of caregivers. The levels of stress, the isolation and the despair point in that direction.

EXERCISE:

1. You must move—dance to DVDs, go up and down the stairs an extra 20 times a day or do simple step aerobics. If an exercise bike or a treadmill or an elliptical trainer is an option, try it out. If walking or running outside is possible and you have the coverage, do that. I usually exercised outside because I live in Southern California where the weather cooperates and I had pretty regular paid help. I used this time to listen to books on the iPod and to talk with family and friends on the phone. Measure your time walking or stair climbing and log it.

2. You must maintain your "core." Work on your abdominal muscles, using basic exercises like crunches and leg lifts. Get on your hands and knees and arch your back. Lie on your back and roll your spine, lifting your hips off the floor. When you are sitting or standing, stretch your shoulders together, toward the front and toward the back. This should feel really good.

3. Integrate simple exercises into your nursing routines. While I stood bedside, feeding my husband, I held in my stomach or did controlled breathing. Filling a water jug at the fridge or standing at the stove, I stood on one leg, working on balance. Unloading the dryer or the dishwasher, I stretched my legs and back.

Moving, core work, stretching and balancing will go a good way toward maintaining "caregiver fitness." Just resist the temptation to think that the unremitting, grinding hard work of grueling nursing care is healthy exercise!

It's also a really good idea to find a personal physician, a doctor, for yourself who understands your situation and has genuine compassion. Such a good doctor will support your efforts at self-care and not give you a hard time when you simply cannot take off those ten pounds or get in for a routine test.

"Chronic Disaster"

What's "chronic" is continuous, unremitting, ongoing. There is no end, certainly no positive end, in sight. What's chronic is somehow manageable. Heart disease, diabetes, cancer, neurological diseases are deemed "manageable." You do this and that, take this and that, and slog on.

What was once unimaginable becomes daily living. So, for some, terrible pain is simply the norm. Others adjust to the horror of amputations. Dementia patients and those who love them somehow cope with awful grief and loss. Individually, caregivers learn the ropes of dialysis, chemotherapy, ventilation—and cheer their loved ones through the pain and sorrow of dependency.

We tend to think of "disaster" as violent and distressing but somehow as a narrative. Think of hurricanes and the shapes on the map on TV. Think of earthquakes, the Richter scale and the violence and the aftershocks. Then come the rescues, the grieving, the funerals, the resolution. There's a beginning, a middle, an end.

Just so, in life and on TV medical shows, we have symptoms, a diagnosis, a treatment (or perhaps a number of treatments), followed by either a cure or failure. On TV it takes just an hour, with time left for staff romance and resentment, subplots and advertisements.

The big diseases, as they are manageable, are chronic and they are disastrous. As disastrous as tornadoes and floods, fires and earthquakes.

They redefine who you are and reshape every aspect of your daily life. They require as much compassionate assistance and they call up what's heroic and wonderful in people—both victims and caregivers and concerned bystanders.

Perhaps there's a useful truth in the idea that some disasters are ongoing, continuous. There's no end in sight. The experience is something that you simply have to get used to, seizing what enjoyment you can, riding with it. The oxymoron of "chronic disaster" betrays a truth about life. The human condition is ongoing, not shaped into segments with resolutions or lessons. We must live in the moment.

Communication

My husband's loss of speech was a gradual thing. For five or six months he needed to be on the "bipap" machine for progressively longer and longer periods. The bipap supported his breathing when his diaphragm failed. The mask that came with the machine covered his mouth. I shopped online for "nasal" masks that pumped air into his nose, freeing his mouth for speech. He became adept at speaking with the bipap and even preached two or three sermons, speaking with each exhalation.

Then his first bout of pneumonia hit. Because he couldn't cough, couldn't clear any mucus from his chest, this was understandable. Agonizing but understandable. When he was intubated he could no longer speak. The next step would be the tracheostomy.

He could still move his facial muscles and, after the intubation, invented an ingenious communication system based on the keypad of a cellphone. The basic grid allowed him to spell words, each letter requiring only two or three or four twitches of his eyebrow. There were three rows, the first row held two boxes, each containing three letters. The second row held three boxes, each containing three letters. The third row contained three boxes as well—the first with p, q, r, s, the second with t, u, and v, the third with w, x, y, and z.

We became very adept with this system, which served us well for the next year, until Gary lost all muscle movement in his face. To read his message, I would ask "Row 1?" no response meant "No, not row one."

Row 2? A raised eyebrow meant "Yes, row two." "Box 1?" A raised eyebrow meant "Yes, box one." "G"—no response. "H"—no response. "I"—and the eyebrow shot up. I would ask "Do you love me?" and the eyebrow shot up—unless he had something else on his mind, of course. So an "F" usually meant the fan. A "U" was a request for the urinal.

Much more sustained communication was also possible. I hired a "secretary" who spent hours taking "dictation" using the system. Letters, sermons, reflections poured from the eyebrow. I would even receive emails at the office.

The loss of the ability to communicate using this system was the most bitter loss of all. We tried various brainwave technologies but none of them worked—or I was too impatient or too limited to make them work.

It was surprising to me how unwilling hospital staff and even friends were to learn the simple system. Hospitals preferred their very primitive poster cartoon diagrams. One lady visitor thought we should all learn Morse code and came supplied with worksheets.

Customer Service

It is no surprise that the quality of telephone "customer service" varies widely. The best customer service is provided by businesses who don't already have your business. Call as a prospective customer and you will be treated respectfully and efficiently. If you have money to spend you will not be put on hold.

If, on the other hand, your insurance is paying for supplies or durable medical equipment (DME), expect to be abused. Apria, a large, national chain, was the worst in this department. If I had a question or if the wrong product had been delivered I would be placed on hold three or four times, totaling as many as 30 minutes. Everybody was busy taking care of other clients—and of course I was supposed to understand.

Waiting on hold is a real burden to a caregiver. An alarm can go off or it's time for a meal or a medication or a turn. Somebody may be at the door or there may be an urgent email to attend to. The business doesn't care. They have you in a stranglehold.

The same suppliers send ridiculously misguided bills—requiring another call, another long wait. They are capable of overnighting two gauze pads in an envelope at ruinous expense. (Some dope confused the code for gauze pads with the code for boxes of gauze pads.)

The same sadistic suppliers enjoy the awful torment of the robo-call. If you are due for a delivery, they will have the computer call your home at some random time, usually interrupting a bowel program or a bath. If you don't push the designated button, as instructed, you risk your supply order being cancelled. If you do push the designated button you are put on hold until the customer service representative has time to take your call!

D

Diagnosis and Disease

This entry is about taking medical science for what it's worth. It's about the actual tentativity of what may be delivered with absolute certainty and authority.

The body is a sacred mystery. Much more is unknown and uncertain than is transparent.

Numbers on laboratory tests and on monitors are only a guide to good care. They are often simply wrong and it has taken years for me not to stress at a low reading or a high reading when the particular device may be on the fritz. So a cold finger yields a dangerously low oxygen saturation. Blood pressure cuffs may go bad or the need for batteries does not register. Rectal probes measuring body temperature can simply not register—and a fever mount without any record. (You may tell the nurse your patient is hot to the touch, even bring in a thermometer. She remains loyal to her machine. You raise a fuss and the thing finally gets "red-tagged." Confidence in the machines continues.)

But it's not just the measuring devices and protocols. I am very unsure about the categories and degrees of disease.

Medical doctors, certainly, are trained to diagnose illnesses and project a future of treatment or irremediable decline. Or perhaps they have less self-confidence than they are trained to project? Perhaps it is the patients and their families who want the certainty of a diagnosis and a prognostication.

For me and for my family, diagnosis is a very iffy business. The perfect confidence of a doctor is an annoying obstacle to good care. The best doctors are open-minded.

So, many years ago, an endocrinologist declared with perfect confidence that our daughter had "premature, irreversible menopause" and would never conceive children. She and her husband have since produced five lovely children without any fertility assistance. This is not really a miracle but rather a useful testimony to the inadequacy of medical diagnosis and prognostication.

So, a highly regarded orthopedic surgeon assured my husband and me that 95 percent of his symptoms could be ascribed to a complicated collapse of one of his vertebrae. Five hours of surgery and Gary never walked again. One neurologist suggested ALS but never performed the requisite tests (muscle biopsy, nerve biopsy, spinal tap). When, finally, another neurologist performed the tests, he found contraindications to any such diagnosis. (The UCLA lab lost the muscle biopsy.)

So a veterinarian once assured us the cat was dying. She lived another couple of years without the feline dialysis at a faraway veterinary school that was supposed to be the only solution.

The worst of it is that patients and family invest the words of a diagnosing MD with terrible authority. It's almost impossible to resist doing this. The weight of these words is one of the many burdens of time in the hospital. Six times we were sent home to die. Eventually the prophecy came true, of course, but it should not have been hung like a pall over our lives.

I understand that much of this is insurance-driven. Certain benefits attach to certain diagnoses. And I have learned to game the system when the anticipation of imminent death is the way to enhanced benefits. But I never put Gary on "hospice," which would have compromised needed treatments and hopeful possibilities.

Dire Moments and Acute Frustrations

Human Nature

I have come to believe that, to a perfectly horrible extent, it is human nature to blame the victim of any catastrophe. Of course this is as old as Job. (Job's friends are certain that he has done something terrible to deserve God's punishment and that just so he must identify his sin and repent.)

Jonathan Swift, in his Verses on the Death of Dr. Swift revisits this idea in dark comic fashion. The reportedly dead Dean is responsible for his reported death—he never took advice.

This came home to me most clearly when, having been ignored for six months by the members and leaders of the church my husband served faithfully before he became ill, I finally asked for a bit of care, a visit. I contacted a co-worker of my husband's, the head of the pre-school. She acted distressed on my behalf and asked if she should bring somebody else along. I suggested the vice president of the congregation accompany her, a woman who had entertained us in her home many times, a woman I had thought of as an upstanding caring Christian exemplar.

They came, with flowers. They spoke to Gary. They spoke to me. And I, desperate and alone, abandoned by all the people who had promised their support and good will, cried out. I said how sad I was and how disappointed that the church had failed us so markedly. I said I was angry.

In return, I was lectured firmly and even cruelly. Told that nobody would visit if I expressed anger or hurt. When I answered that nobody had called or visited for many months so I had never had a chance to express these things, I was told that just that attitude was the problem.

So I was to blame. And they never came back. And we were, for the most part, on our own. Those were the good Christians, the church ladies, the representatives of a community of love.

One Awful Night

In those six years the most awful night of all was at a poor-quality hospital in Los Angeles where the ambulance had taken Gary when he started to fade away with what turned out to be pneumonia. He had been intubated, then extubated and put back on the bipap (external breathing machine) and then, after two or three weeks, released from the ICU to a regular ward. He had devised the communication system and communicated to me that something was very wrong. I went to the charge nurse and told her. She said they would give him a tranquilizer. I asked if his neurologist had approved the tranquilizer—a major concern. I said that he was agitated because he couldn't breathe. She said there was an order for Ativan. It was the middle of the night. I called the miserable ICU doctor and managed to kick the system into action. An ER doctor rushed into the room. I was thrown out. Last view I had was of the ER doctor, straddling Gary, intubating him once again. I graded papers for an hour in the waiting room while Gary struggled for life. When his oxygen levels were normal we were returned to the ICU where the saga continued.

Panic Attack

From my notes:

Gary's fever still hasn't topped 101, even when the Tylenol has worn off, so I shouldn't panic. But oh my, the awful experience of septic shock last month weighs constantly on my mind. So many terrors. So many scares. So much terrible news. His fracture, the leg broken months ago and never caught, is very much with me. I simply cannot protect him or prevent disasters. All I can do is wait, measure, react. This is wearing me down. The long stretches of stability are healing, certainly, but right now I don't know if we're there or on our way into another pit.

Sorting It All Out
Spent the entire day on Medicare issues.

Here's the point: Medicare says they'll cover 28-35 hours per week of home health care for Gary. The church (i.e., employers') disability advisors agree. Requirements (for him) are a breeze. I have this from two supervisors and a half dozen customer service people at Medicare.

The issue is that I cannot find a single Medicare-certified home health agency that agrees that Medicare will pay for anything more than token "assessment" visits! I have contacted at least 10 agencies. Even the Cedars-Sinai home coordinator insists that Medicare won't pay for home health care—despite the published documents and websites that are very clear!

One agency administrator (at "Best Care" in Santa Monica) simply declared that "Medicare won't pay."

Now the sweet guy at Medicare (David Berger) could only think of one solution—I should go to the State Medical Certification people and go after the agencies as certified by the State! Seems a huge tangle to just get that to which we are entitled!

If this is indeed the case, then tens of thousands of people in the LA area entitled to home care have been deprived by a network of agencies that either don't understand the benefits OR have decided it's too much hassle to provide the benefits and misrepresent Medicare.

Update: In San Diego, not in Los Angeles, Medicare pays for three baths and two RN visits per week.

Trach(eostomy) Tubing

From my notes:

When I came home yesterday afternoon I found Leslie concerned that she couldn't find the "cushion" attached to Gary's trach tube. The cushion is a signal system, a little balloon, attached by a narrow tube, to the "cuff" that holds the trach tube in place. I found it, totally flat, in the "trach collar" that holds the trach tube in place.

I tried to inflate the cushion, which one fills with air via a special syringe. It wouldn't fill. This meant that the cuff was somehow leaking. Sure enough, air was escaping from the trachea, around the tube, resulting in bubbling from Gary's nose and mouth.

I thought perhaps we could make it through the night and Mariana could replace the tube in the morning. I know that some people use "cuffless trach tubes," which means that air escapes all the time and it's ok. But the alarm kept sounding, so I had to decide around 8:30 pm that I would change the tube myself, then.

I have never before changed a trach tube. For more than three years now I have watched. I have been tutored. I have taught caregivers how to do it. But the actual process has always worried me, worried me that I would pass out—killing Gary as a result. There is something so very taboo about pushing a plastic device into the hole in the throat of a beloved husband. I know too well that many mothers and fathers do this regularly to their "trached" babies and little children. You do what you have to do. An early ENT (Ear, Nose and Throat) MD brushed off my horror. I remained steadfast in my terror.

Nevertheless, having celebrated the end of my semester with a couple of vodka and cranberry juice drinks, I opened Gary's eyes and told him what we were going to do, called Leslie in for support, put on a pair of sterile gloves, and proceeded:

We raised the lower half of the bed and, using the draw sheet, pulled Gary to the top of his bed. I removed his pillow and put a foam neck roll behind his neck and raised the head of the bed.

I opened the box with the new tube and tested the inflation system to make certain that this tube wasn't defective as well. Everything seemed in order and the cuff inflated as I injected air, then deflated when I extracted the air. I removed the "inner cannula" from the tube and replaced it with the "obdurator," a curved projectile that smoothes the leading edge of the tube so that it passes easily into the hole and then into the trachea.

Leslie removed the trach collar and the dressings and then, on my count, pulled the trach tube.

The hole was, as always, a violent and terrible, gaping thing to me. I pushed the tube into the hole—there is always some resistance. I extracted the obdurator and replaced it with the inner cannula (which it took me a very long 2 seconds to find, wrapped in sterile plastic but under a fold in the bedding). Leslie quickly reattached the ventilator circuit and Gary's chest rose and fell with fresh breath.

I inflated the cuff of the new trach tube, we tucked in the new dressing and connected a new collar to hold the whole thing in place.

The low pressure alarm never sounded, which meant that the whole procedure had taken only seconds. A quick wave of nausea had to be from the adrenaline.

The high pressure alarm stopped its nagging and both Gary and I were comfortable for the rest of the evening and through the night.

Disability

We chose consistently to use the language of "disability" rather than "disease." Total, speechless paralysis is certainly acute disability—and it was less scary for all of us, especially the little children, than the language of disease. This was assuredly a disability caused by disease—the death of all Gary's motor neurons driving his skeletal muscles. But it was not a contagious condition or something to be feared.

The idea of disability also preserves human integrity. The whole person remains here with us, albeit not able to walk or speak, to gesture or move. The high heroic models of Stephen Hawking and Christopher Reeve are available and useful.

It was hard to do the paperwork for Social Security disability and a kind friend did most of it for me. (Thank you, John Rollefson.) I wasn't ready but the benefits were important. The inexorable progression of the disability was less painful for me in the months that followed than the inexorable loss of benefits!

(As I have noted, my husband's employer used his condition as a warrant for dumping him into Medicare—which covers certain neurological conditions in people under 65—and stripping him of his employer-provided health insurance. Just so, he could be forcibly removed from disability benefits and "retired" at a much lesser income when he turned 66.)

E

Energy (Good and Bad):

From my notes:

I found myself this morning getting unreasonably annoyed at the nurse who, yesterday, put medical trash from changing out Gary's catheter in the fancy garbage bags I order online to fit the fancy Simple Human garbage can. (These bags cost, maybe, eight cents, and take, maybe, 60 seconds to order in bulk every few months.) How could she be so unthinking? So wasteful? I noticed that another caregiver—an equally kind and generous heart—put a Nutren (formula for tube feeding) can and a small cardboard carton in the trash rather than the recycling! How could she be so dense, so unobservant after all these weeks? The cans and boxes always go into the recycling! Didn't I make that clear?

In the days before Gary's disability I regularly had help with the cleaning. I never stressed the small stuff. I have always resented my own mother's control over details of household economy. Am I becoming my mother?

I don't think so. I am very tired today from working too hard yesterday and waking up long before dawn, still buzzed, perhaps, on adrenaline. Is it my tiredness speaking? I don't think so.

Is it some pathetic cry for control in a life spun out of control—a life in which I cannot leave the house because the caregivers this week aren't trustworthy with the finer points of life support? But I'm getting lots done, the house is pretty and the garden blooming and I had wonderful visits from family last weekend and expect more soon.

I think my cranky judgmentalism was simply sin—on a small scale, of course, but that's how sin picks at a beautiful, hopeful day. Sin may be funny in retrospect, but at the time it is gnat-like in its annoyance. There's no way to swat it back. It hums and buzzes and bites. I'm annoyed at people who help me, impatient and miserly over a nickel's worth of value.

I'm not about to beat myself up about something so inconsequential—growing the gnat sin into a monster. But that it even occurred is a reminder of my weakness and vulnerability.

I may be tired. I told one of the grandsons that I felt old. He said, forthrightly and appropriately, "You *are* old!" Of course. But I'm supposed to maintain my energy, exercise and take vitamins. I have a huge home to maintain, a staff of half a dozen caregivers, long lists of business tasks—suppliers, insurers, medical offices. And there are dozens of half-finished writing projects waiting in piles and in files. How can I do all this work if I'm old and tired? AND walk five miles a day!

I read in pop spirituality texts online and in occasional student papers about good energy and bad energy. Indeed, the language of energy complicates our already intricate daily lives. How much of good energy is the same smiley face cheerfulness that is savaged in so much criticism of the moronic face of the fifties housewife?

It has new forms and manifestations. I seem to have subscribed to a website that puts bits of advice in my inbox every few days—advising me to garden, to breathe in this or that way, to cleanse, to fast, to go for long walks, to find a good source of local organic produce, to fill my home with flowers. The list is endless. The life of total loveliness and simple pleasure-seeking—and, in the end, self-absorption—is alluring. Surely this would be an invigorating (i.e. energizing) way to live, slim and spacey, calm and orderly. Ahhh.

A dying actress friend wanted to expel all bad energy from her home, her space, her body. I asked her if that meant I should not visit as my energy was, at least to me, to the extent I understood the concept, suspicious. I am critical, questioning rather than accepting just about everything. I am restless and often sarcastic! I am often fiercely angry. These just may be bad energy, hardly zen. They have me calling to complain and supporting this cause or that.

What's worse, I live and breathe sickness and death. Nurses and suppliers, most doctors and technicians shake their heads in front of me or behind my back, convinced that I am deluded or lost. When we are in a hospital, the bad energy drapes us, that pall.

At home, I am up to my elbows in the contamination of bowel programs and mucus and pressure sores. There's stink there, and germs and slime. I am fouled, unclean, polluted by any standards I know of from my work in women and global religions. I deal in dirty towels and dirty bed linen, dirty gauze and murky tubes and disposable this and that. This cannot possibly make for good energy! And I can upset myself over somebody else's choice of garbage bags or bins! That's bad.

What's clean and orderly, gleaming and sweet-smelling, bright and cheery, that's good. But it's only one side and to see it requires turning away from the whole world of woe.

Evaluations

A few days after every return from the hospital, I would check the mail and there they'd be—the batch of evaluations from the hospital. One was about the emergency room. One was about the balance of the hospital stay—nurses, doctors, food, housekeeping. Now we all are asked to fill out such forms all the time. EBay sellers, Amazon experiences, daily living seems to require constant feedback, poured into multiple choice forms with room for comment.

I used to ignore the forms from hospitals. My hands were more than full and my days terribly long as my beloved husband was struggling to recover and was hardly stable. (What passes for stable in the hospital—and ready for discharge—isn't quite yet home care stable.) But the nurses I spoke with had insisted that these forms were really important for the hospital ratings and standings.

So I opened the forms. No problem with the ER document. Everything was great. We were treated promptly and well. Of course when a white male and his rather commanding wife appear in an ambulance, when the patient is on a ventilator already, they don't stick you in a waiting room. Triage dictates you move to the head of the line. The dozens of brown people and their concerned families hunched in the waiting room are passed by. (It's called triage but it seems unfair nonetheless.) We were treated very well, very promptly. Our own doctor even showed up after an hour or so. There was a long wait for a bed, but there are only a few beds set up for ventilators and hospital time has its own groove.

The questionnaire about the hospital stay was seriously troubling, however. How to "grade" the nursing care? During a month-long stay we were cared for by at least 30 different nurses, working 12-hour shifts. Some were one-shift nurses. Others returned repeatedly. Some were highly competent but not very cordial. Others were very personable but made mistakes or failed to show up when needed. Twice-daily evaluations might have been more accurate, but they would have been a terrible hassle. To grade the nursing care in a lump was simply impossible!

Caution: as an educator, I have graded for a living. Countless grades, weekly, midterm, final. I have written scores of letters of recommendation for students, for colleagues, for friends. I should be good at these sorts of assessments, but they make me simply crazy. Bad nurses shouldn't be allowed to compromise the scores of good nurses. Long hospital stays should allow for detailed and comprehensive evaluation, but the assessment forms don't permit that. Who better to provide feedback than a spouse who has been to many hospitals, who spends six or eight hours bedside each day, who knows the details of complex nursing care from years of providing and overseeing it at home?

But these primitive forms disallow any such evaluation and seem more like a survey of hotel satisfaction.

And what of the doctors? Some failed utterly to communicate. (If I wasn't present at the random time, unannounced, they made their rounds I was simply uninformed.) Other doctors were attentive and compassionate. How could I grade their collective competence? Did they get top marks because my husband had survived the stay? Was that good and sufficient recommendation?

F

Finding Fault

Lamentably, much of nursing seems poisoned by fault-finding. Anybody and everybody is to blame for whatever isn't right. Most invidiously, the patient is seen as somehow responsible for his or her plight. (I have listened carefully.) Various bad behaviors lead to cancer and heart disease, so the sufferer is responsible. Disobedience of one sort or another—not taking medicines, not following instructions, not getting a second opinion, not consulting this or that specialist or having this or that test all are the victim's fault. So a distraught caregiver who doesn't exercise or eat vegetables or who does drink too much or does get angry is, on one or another level, guilty and so deserving of whatever misery awaits.

This is often unconscious. The motive is the need for relief—from the pressing anxiety that if I don't smoke or don't get fat, if I get the tests and do everything I'm told, then I certainly will never end up in this condition. Blaming behaviors provides an explanation for the suffering and the grief, letting the whole towering reality of suffering and death loom in a fog of righteous assurance.

But it's not just the physical blame. A patient with no visitors is presumed to have been an unpleasant person, understandably abandoned by family and friends. The unpleasantness is palpable in the hospital, where the victim of such neglect may curse and groan, struggle against restraints and be a real handful.

Nurses also find fault with one another. Long shifts and terrible responsibilities contribute to a culture of fault-finding. So the nameless nurse on the prior shift did a bad job changing a dressing or didn't keep accurate records or failed in some other way. So I may impugn the skills of one nurse to ingratiate myself with another. I may do this in all innocence—asking questions about a standard of care—or with a measure of malice, truly sensing neglect or indifference.

There's a fine line between the righteous complaint about hygiene or mistakes (wrong medication or wrong schedule, defective measurements or failure to appear altogether) and minor fault-finding. The poison air hangs everywhere.

G

Giving up

It's not right to give up. But not giving up has to be held in perfect balance with level-headed clarity. This balance is a moral and an intellectual and a spiritual discipline. I suspect many of the millions who share my situation, or a similar situation, share this experience.

As long as there is life there is hope. This is not a delusional but a faithful hope. God is great and good and Jesus, the incarnate Lord, healed the sick and even raised the dead. To despair is to deny the greatness and the goodness and the providence of God and the care, compassion and power of Jesus Christ. That denial is too dark for words. That despair is worse than any imaginable loss.

Many of us had friends with AIDS who gave up in the months before the drug cocktails appeared that turned AIDS into a chronic, rather than a terminal, condition. Science may yet provide a fix for neuromuscular disease. Engineering may provide a means of communication through "brain computer interface" technology or BCI. Or, probably, not. All of life is uncertain. We knew that.

Many visitors and friends, even family members, failed to understand. They wanted to mourn with me, lament all the losses: He was so strong, so loving, so brilliant. Such an athlete! Such a pastor! Such a leader! The time for mourning and lamentation would certainly come, but it wasn't yet there and the grief and sorrow were premature. Indeed, grieving threw off the crucial, sane balance of the moment.

In one later hospitalization, this came home especially clearly when a nurse asked about Gary, "Was he a Lakers fan?" I reported her to her supervisor. To refer to somebody who is living in the past tense is a gross mistake. It is untrue to the situation and a bad reflection of the sort of care one might expect of such a nurse.

But hospitalizations are really hard under the best circumstances. Medical people like to fix things. It's their strength and their awful weakness when faced with situations they can't begin to fix. Usually it's the doctors who can only respond with dire prognostications or depressive glances. The rare, good doctors understand that all we can do is to do what we can, to fix what can be fixed and hope for the best.

To give up hope, to despair, is to lose all the calm focus that allows the daily service of caring for a terribly disabled husband or child or parent. This is true at home as in the hospital.

Of course there is grief here! (Don't be stupid.) Of course there are awful losses! When I would think that it had been four or five long years since my husband and lover could speak my name—and that even then it was gaspingly, spacing out his words through the bipap—when I recalled the lovely baritone of his voice, I could not hold back the tears. For years I avoided the street that passed by the hospital in Los Angeles where he was tracheostomized, where, like the Little Mermaid, he left his voice. (We kept his cell phone account for years because the voicemail message was a precious chance to hear his voice. He was permanently "unable to answer our call.")

His huge wheelchair was a monument in space to his awful, total paralysis.

Certainly his wasted body, his protruding tongue, his bedsores were all reminders of the wages of his disease.

But please, let's not be maudlin or teary. That doesn't help. And if you want to be supportive of those of us who are coping with a long-term, awful chronic disability, family and friends, co-workers and clergy must avoid laying their grief at our door, for us to clean up. Help came from visitors and friends who were willing to speak to my husband, to tell him about their worlds, their kids, their hopes and their sorrows. This broke the silence and took him out of his bed and into fresh spaces. Help came from those who intuited that we needed distraction.

I sought for all those years not to be pathetic! Tragic was OK, so long as you brought humor and grace, not tears, into my home. But to be pathetic is to lose all standing, all promise, all grown up humanity. You may pity us and you may fear for yourselves—as susceptible to awful disease as we are—such pity and fear are, according to Aristotle, the essence of tragedy. You may recall that we were important people, powerful and charismatic. That enhances the pity and the fear. It's required. But don't cancel out our living, breathing selves with the pathos that obscures the sufferer.

And please, don't make me share my struggles! Such a common question—And how are YOU doing? I think this is well-intentioned, but you really don't want to know! You want, rather, an answer that will let you report—"She is so strong!" or "She's really falling apart!" The experience is so intricate, so complicated, that sharing where I am is not really possible in any such conversation.

Nor did I need to vent, to share my feelings, thank you very much. My subjectivity remained intact, my sanity preserved, because of boundaries and perspective. To vent was to lose control. Control was essential under those circumstances.

(Do, by all means, find competent professional help if and when you need it! Good therapists are out there and some are especially skilled in just this sort of support.)

So what is a friend to do? I think that normal social intercourse is the key. We can talk about grandchildren or vacations, about books and articles. There are so many experiences to report, so many impressions and ideas. Friends can bring normalness into a terribly difficult situation.

Normalness matters hugely. When every breath is mechanically managed, every calorie pumped through a tube, every book and periodical downloaded onto an iPod and powered directly into the brain, when every outing takes an hour to prepare and every bowel movement is an elaborate and ugly process—under such circumstances, normal is pure grace.

I have for years now been sure that many people didn't approve of us and second-guessed our choices. There were the little things, of course, like obstructing traffic with the wheelchair van when I had to slow down because the alarm on the vent was sounding, or ramps that banged and doubtless annoyed the neighbors. But I am sure, unreasonably sure, that church people were annoyed by our electrical cords and the wheezing of the vent during the service. I am sure they resented having to walk around the huge chair, semi-reclined. I'm sure some thought it was obscene to bring somebody so strange-looking into church.

I suspect that many people have suggested it would have been better all around to "pull the plug" or otherwise to end Gary's suffering. That he was evidently not suffering, just being the best he could be, a heroic fighter, didn't fit their convictions. They wanted us to give up!

H

Hiring Help—and Letting Go

In my experience, self-identified home care providers have ample skills—in bathing and, sometimes, massage, in dressing and grooming, in turning and in wound care. They have training of one sort or another and experience and few have ever done anything egregious or dangerous when I have hired them myself. (Agency workers are not so certain.)

As a group however, most care providers lack the basic ability to make good use of the down time that goes with the job. For many hours of a work day, after basic care, there is just not much to do—except the hourly turning and constant readiness for a serious emergency. "My" patient is sleeping or listening to books, perhaps watching television. Or a visitor has stopped by to pass the time.

It can be lonely work. When other help was around—a housecleaner or a phlebotomist or visiting nurse—I saw how a care provider would light up and engage in conversation. In a "facility," where the work is arduous and incessant—bathing and dressing a dozen patients or more during a shift—the labor is relieved by camaraderie and the presence of coworkers is a pleasure.

Home care is another story, especially home care of patients silenced by stroke or neuromuscular failure, patients suffering from dementia or the comatose.

I learned to mention this when I interviewed prospective helpers. How do they fill the quiet hours? Do they read or knit? I provided a laptop with Wi-Fi for workers who were students. I tried to chat—although my own work agenda was fairly strict. Some spent hours texting or on their cell phones. One helper was setting up a production company—and couriers delivered movie scripts to the front door.

If somebody skilled wasn't available, I would hire a kind, able-bodied, teachable person. The aspiring producer had no training and she was very good.

I learned to do every task any nurse or caregiver performed, from the lowliest to the most technical. This gave me credibility and even authority and made for better relationships with caregivers. But I preferred to have a seasoned worker train a new worker, largely because that improved the self-esteem of the practiced helper.

Care providers burn out. They move on. A year is about the most you can expect. Their lives are often full of stress and pressure and parents or grown kids suddenly find themselves in a jam and need your care provider to come back home. This is likely a pretext and in fact the job—however pleasant the space and comfortable the situation—gets old.

Signs of burnout may include rudeness and anger. One nurse, otherwise a gem, as she moved out, wrote a very hurtful letter, declaring that I was killing my husband with my bad care and neglect. Another stopped speaking to me almost entirely and left without saying goodbye. ("Patsy" stormed out in a fury. See Rogues Gallery, below). Rarely do these kind and generous people understand that they have burned out. They are just unhappy and angry and confused.

Hospital Care

When we were in the hospital, I would talk with nurses because it helped pass the time, because they were interesting people, because they were interested in my life with my husband. I sometimes suspected that I also talked with nurses, respiratory therapists, even technicians and cleaning staff, because I sensed that they would be more helpful, take more care, be more attentive and considerate if they understood me, my husband, my children and grandchildren.

I wanted them to love us!

I don't know if this is normal, but I think that patients who are attended by family members are more highly regarded than those who are alone. And the more constantly they are attended, the more carefully they will be managed by hospital staff. This isn't fair, of course, and it places a terrific burden on the families of patients, but it's only human for hospital staff to invest more in those who are clearly important to others.

Patients who are shampooed and shaven, whose skin is well-cared for, who smell good and whose eyes are clear are better treated. They are respected. The same rules apply, lamentably, to the ill as to the well. Grooming matters. Nevertheless, in hospitals nobody washes the hair of the bed-bound. They may provide nasty "shampoo caps" that allow for "waterless washing," but these leave hair stringy and badly scented. (Anybody who suggests their use should be sentenced to four weeks of washing her own hair using only the occasional shampoo cap.)

My husband watched television. At home he had a huge plasma screen and a headset that raised the volume to a level he could hear over the whoosh of the ventilator, breathing into his throat. To set him up to watch TV, I would hold his eyes open with a stretchy headband, put his glasses on and position his head just so. Then I stood in front of the screen to make sure his eyes were exactly aligned and focused. In the hospital, where the TV was way up high, this involved standing on a chair.

After a nurse had seen Gary watching TV she was usually much more engaged, much more compassionate, much less likely to write him off as comatose or a humanoid vegetable.

Gail Collins in a useful column a number of years ago dealt with this desire to charm, to ingratiate the hospital staff treating a beloved brother. She thought back to the hospital-acquired infection that ultimately cost his life and about how often she saw hospital staff come into the room without washing their hands or putting on gloves, about how she never told them to wash up, fearful that they would take offense and treat her brother less well. I think she was picking up on a very human tendency of all people to want to ingratiate those upon whom we depend, those who hold the powers of pain and comfort, death and life, in their hands.

Hospital Communication

I learned from hard experience that if I really wanted to get through to a hospital staff with requests and instructions, I needed to fax the nursing station. I had to type a firm but deferential letter with my list of concerns and fax it in. Such faxes become part of a patient's working file and are treated with great respect.

Calls, cries, appeals that are undocumented are only sometimes heard by a single nurse or charge nurse.

Just so, smartphone pictures of egregious mistakes and bad practices, of untreated sores or rashes, carry particular weight. They are against the rules, of course, but they are easy to take and a source of power to the patient.

Hospital Discharge/Going Home

Discharge is the great goal of a hospital stay. It's graduation from what was and commencement of a new chapter of life at home. There's relief and hopefulness, of course. Relief from the grind of hospital routine and new faces and bad news and blood tests and monitors and hope that home will be a place of healing and calm and friendliness.

But there's fear as well. What will we do when nurses and doctors are no longer close by? Even for a caregiver as practiced as I became, hospital stays were disabling. As the days went by, my husband was more and more medicalized. While he may have been overcoming an infection, xrays and MRIs and various electrocardiograms always seemed to have revealed medical anomalies, little things that might indicate big things.

As he was more medicalized, my confidence would shrink, my can-do mentality flag.

Years ago, with the early discharges, officious "discharge planners" managed everything—but they clearly weren't very savvy. I remember one lady questioning whether insurance would pay for an ambulance trip home—of a totally paralyzed patient on a ventilator! I got the van and the chair and took my husband home myself. (At that same fancy Beverly Hills hospital a "transfer" from bed to wheelchair meant a very large, sumo wrestler type man lifting my 6'4" husband in his arms and heaving him into the wheelchair.)

Discharge planners normally release patients to rehabilitation, where insurance pays for weeks of—mostly poor-quality—care. They are ignorant about home care and promise resources they can't deliver and provide quantities of "durable medical equipment" of questionable value. The guidelines seem to be what insurance will pay for rather than what a particular patient actually needs.

The discharge may also include training, training you to care for your loved one at home. Such training is probably the worst of the bad experiences I have had in the whole history of caring for my husband. I never expected a short course in practical nursing, but thought that basic tasks like cleaning of the tracheostomy site could be explained and demonstrated with kindness and precision.

Hospital Nightmares

In a number of the hospitals and "facilities" where I spent many weeks, I observed in horror the terrible one-upmanship that prevails. The hierarchy is absolute and authoritarian and chillingly inappropriate in a workplace dedicated to giving care. The lofty specialists appear unannounced and unscheduled. The only way to be sure to speak with one of these superior beings is to remain at bedside 24/7. The staff doctors are somewhat more available, although well shielded by the nursing staff, protected from patient or family questions. The charge nurse models her role on the staff doctors, spending her day behind a computer terminal at the nurses' desk. The nurse assigned to patients also spends many hours at the computer. Most are harried and angry when they are interrupted. The lower-level nurses—practical nurses and certified nursing assistants—are generally very touchy about who does what. God forbid you should ask a nurse for something a CNA is supposed to provide or report to a CNA that the floor is very dirty! Respiratory therapists and other technicians are similarly jealous of their tasks and unavailable for any other duties.

It gets even nastier in large urban hospitals where the staff is largely foreign-born—African, Asian, Latin American, Pacific Islander. The pecking order and authority issues from a dozen countries all converge. Language problems abound. Many nurses have doubtless mastered scientific English but their grasp of conversational English is tenuous. They say rude and terrible things! They misunderstand questions and, almost entirely, miss any nuance.

One important task of hospital staff is to teach skills to family members who will be caring for their patient at home. Often these "teachers" are the evident products of a teaching-learning environment that is condescending and judgmental and sees no value in positive reinforcement or encouragement.

I had to learn to clean around the new, raw hole in my beloved husband's neck, the "tracheostomy site." This was disturbing for me, almost sick-making. I was instructed in the procedure by half a dozen different nurses, each with a brusque manner and a heavy accent. Each one did the procedure differently. Each one condemned me roundly for doing the job exactly as the former nurse-teacher had. My protests were brushed aside. Nobody understood my horror or offered any comfort or reassurance.

Hospital Nurses

Nurses in a modern hospital seem to be a strange hybrid of blue collar service worker and highly trained technical professional.

I have thought a lot about the hospital pecking order. In some hospitals, the innocent patient or spouse who asks for fresh linen or notes a dirty floor had better be really careful not to imply that a nurse is responsible. Housekeeping should be notified, but via channels. Just so, if a patient needs respiratory therapy, don't ask the wrong nurse or you will be reprimanded. (Most nurses do, however, like to hear complaints about doctors.)

I have spent many hours talking with nurses. They are mostly really interesting people. Many seem to live lives of terrible stress (although that may be California-specific). They are transient and have lived in many places. Their marriages seem to me, on average, less stable than community norms. Some have lost children to drugs. Many have cared for elderly parents. They seem to like working 12-hour shifts because of the freedom that comes from long stretches of free time but, as the hours drag on, the strain is often visible and attention flags. (It would be interesting to compare the responsiveness to calls, the frequency of errors, the accuracy of charting, at 2, 4, 6, 8, 10, and 12 hours.)

Hospital Time

Visiting Hours: I was not a *visitor*! I was my husband's primary caregiver, his advocate, his lifeline. I knew how to make him physically comfortable and how to reassure him. To dismiss me from his bedside so that nurses could do their "assessments" and share their notes during shift change was highhanded. It was not in the best interest of my husband. Hospital protocol calls for more than an hour in the morning and another in the evening when all family and visitors are expelled. Fortunately, this is often negotiable. Good nurses allow continuity of care. If some battle axe doesn't get it, fax the nursing station with your arguments.

Pacing: When we lived in the Caribbean, people, both locals and expat Americans, joked about "Island time." Schedules were impossible. Lives were so subject to contingencies that nobody could be sure to make an appointment and doctors scheduled everybody for 8 am and then just made you wait your turn. Church services and committee meetings began when a good number of people—maybe a quorum but not necessarily—had arrived. Awful traffic, a sudden downpour, a sick or pokey child, a call from a relative, a sudden urgent distraction—any or all of these could disrupt your best plans. And the people you were meeting would understand. They probably had their own challenges and were going to be really late as well.

Large families, pacing from a simpler day, a simple willingness to be late were all factors. Still, students came to class on time, perhaps having been drilled by the nuns in parochial school. Planes left on time, perhaps because of the strictures of the FAA. Not everything went by Island time.

Hospital time reminds me of my years in Puerto Rico. Doctors round whenever it suits them or after the surgery is done for the day. (A favorite neurologist regularly showed up after 10 pm.) Procedures scheduled for one time get put off by half an hour or more, perhaps an emergency, perhaps a traffic jam. A simple transfer or "turn" requires a large cast of characters, the "lift team," some of whom may have left for lunch or gone home. (We once waited over an hour for the lift team to help transfer my husband from the gurney to his wheelchair only to learn that the team was one guy who had gone home, feeling unwell.) There's no contending with the squishiness of hospital time. It's terribly wasteful of staff time and resources. It can be painful for patients and even nurses as they perform lifts or turns without bracing or equipment.

Hygiene

As I don't "believe" in modern scientific medicine, so I don't "believe" in radical antisepsis. Germs are our friends, keeping our immune systems sharp and ingenious.

Nor is life in a bubble appealing. Small children are infested with germs, dripping noses, hacking coughs, dirty hands. But they belong in the space of the chronically ill, for their sakes and for the sake of the patient, for whom their touch and their voices provide transcendent relief. Much better to die of a cold, contracted from the wet kiss of a toddler, than to live without those kisses. Nor is sterile bedding and filtered air a desired end.

Which brings us to the issue of hand washing and gloves. Good hospitals, with good reason, suggest that patients and families help enforce hand-washing. Every staff person, from the lowliest tech to the loftiest specialist is to wash his or her hands when entering the hospital room. Alternatively, fresh gloves or careful use of hand sanitizers is permitted. This is to protect the patient, not the nurse or the doctor, from one of a long list of hospital-contracted infections.

Nevertheless, hospital staff is terribly lax, terribly negligent, terribly confused. Some nurses feel that gloves seem hostile or fearful, that patients think they are sources of contamination. They won't use gloves when they really should and their motives are irreproachable but the result can be the spread of disease. Others are genuinely fearful of a patient's cooties and use gloves to protect themselves—often the same gloves with multiple patients! Hand sanitizers, used carelessly, are no substitute for hand-washing.

So what is reasonable in a home? Like so many decisions, it depends on the individual. Most dangerous, in my experience, are workers who come straight from "facilities" where patients are often warehoused in less-than-ideal circumstances. Three days after one such worker showed up at our home, my husband was rushed to the hospital with a kind of pneumonia that thrives in institutional settings. Ideally, such workers would be required to shower and change clothes before crossing the threshold of a private home. Certainly they should scrub their hands in surgical fashion.

Dopey or simply sleepy nurses require constant vigilance. One miserable nurse came to work in latex gloves—bringing city germs into the house but somehow, in her mind, acting professionally. Just so, "scrubs" are a dubious item of health care when they are worn in restaurants, in the car, on the street.

Bedding should certainly be laundered in warm water, using bleach for anything fouled by feces. Pillows and blankets need regular laundering. We shampooed carpets every two or three months and wiped down surfaces weekly. The dishwasher virtually sterilized canisters and feeding supplies. I kept plenty of gloves on hand and encouraged their use. Most importantly, nobody made it to my husband's bedside without a stop in the powder room for a good hand washing.

I

Identity

So who am I? and who is the one I am caring for?

I am reminded of the stress of being a mom, when, after a long day of hard work, perhaps following a sleepless night, every mother wonders if there's anything left of who she was before having children—the smart, sexy, independent free spirit who could pack her bag in ten minutes and hit the road. Or the husband who misses his bachelor days and the self he cultivated with the help of the ads that play on television during sporting events!

I regularly had to "introduce" my husband to a new caregiver or a nurse in the hospital, or somebody who never knew him when he was able-bodied, eloquent and able to smile. Every time I did so, I rehearsed in my mind not who he had been but who he was still. We must imagine that who we are is the best of who we have been, that our selfhood, our basic humanity, our identity, isn't comprised of what becomes of us in the worst times.

For Christians, this is the self as "saint," as a child of God, as a blessed and beloved creature whose life is under divine care throughout our days. For just about anybody it makes no sense to define ourselves by the worst of times, when we are dirty or sick or crazed with passion or despair.

The staff at a good Alzheimer's unit may acknowledge this by posting a picture of the resident when he or she was in prime shape, along with a biographical sketch. This is the person who is really present, not the shadow, not the cranky and confused old lady.

So the amputee is not defined by his or her present maimed condition but by the runner he or she once was. So the bald and vomiting "victim" is essentially, basically, truly the person she was before the cancer struck. So, over the ventilator at the head of his bed, I hung a huge poster of my husband and a friend in a cave at the top of a cliff to which they had backpacked, carrying 60 pounds of water each. In the photo he is wearing his camping socks, which he wore in bed on cold days after his paralysis.

This is not delusional! Clearly you and I, as caregivers, are perfectly aware of the wages of disease and the reality of paralysis, amputation, silence or dementia. But the fundamental identity of the beloved for whom we care must not be allowed to slip. Lovers and parents know that, certainly. The person one loves is the best imaginable version of him or herself. When love slips and we look for faults and failings, that's catastrophic.

Just so, one's own identity is at stake here. I was never just a wife or just a mother. So I refused to be just a devoted and sacrificial caregiver. My own identity was multiple, variable from day to day, even in my sixties. Indeed, when I overdid it, spending, say, 48 hours without any help, without being able to leave the house, I became practically haunted. The physical labor seemed utterly overwhelming. The loneliness drove me crazy. I lost myself. I had trouble reading or writing, cooking or cleaning, doing anything useful at all. When help arrived at last I fled.

Isolation (Hospital)

At random times during our five hospitalizations of 3-6 weeks over those six years, mysterious test results determined that my husband was carrying an awful infection. There are numbers of such scary infections—all hospital-acquired and all supposedly deadly. One is MRSA, described by the Mayo Clinic site: "Methicillin-resistant Staphylococcus Aureus (MRSA) infection is caused by a strain of staph bacteria that's become resistant to the antibiotics commonly used to treat ordinary staph infections." Symptoms include terrible boils!

Some routine tests found he had no such infections. Others red-flagged him as a carrier. Clearly he was not suffering from a staph infection and clearly he had no boils whatsoever. Nevertheless, suddenly and with great energetic activity, a stack of yellow gowns appeared outside his room and a scary sign was posted on the door: ISOLATION! Now everybody entering the room was to don a gown, gloves, and a mask—which they then discarded in a huge bin by the door.

Now, technically, contamination was a terrible threat to me, my children, my grandchildren, the nurses, the techs, and every patient in the hospital. It was explained to me that if I got on an elevator or went to the cafeteria I risked spreading this plague to other people in other wards and wings of the hospital.

Despite these dire warnings, many nurses and techs came into the room with only cursory attention to such rules. Many doctors skipped the gowns. I watched my husband prepared to be taken for tests by nurses and techs with no gowns. He was wheeled through the halls with no precautions. In the lab nobody wore gowns—indeed I had to yell at a technician who dropped his glove on the floor and then picked it up to put on his hand.

Neither the test nor the protocol make any common sense. In my worst moments I imagined that it was just another way to stress patients and their families. If the threat were serious, surely a modern hospital could muster a more consistent and convincing protocol!

Isolation (Personal)

We all deal with personal isolation. In bed, late at night, unable to contact anybody without scaring them half to death, we are alone. During the day, when we can't get out, the isolation can be terrible. Phone calls and email, Facebook and real, physical visits relieve the isolation. It is, however, a basic fact of life, whether you are caring for a disabled person or whether you are simply alive and needing human contact, that acute loneliness is the norm in certain life stages.

I am aware that extreme neediness is very off-putting, very alienating. Even good friends and family members may recoil in the face of extreme neediness. When it got to be too much to bear, I turned to anti-anxiety medication.

J

Joys

Care is hard but not only hard.

This is a beloved body in your care. Both being cared for and caring for somebody you love is a very sweet thing. Anybody who has ever been fed special food, prepared with love, knows this. If you have been lovingly massaged, you know this from the receiving end. Anybody who has ever shaved her man or given him a pedicure knows this sweetness.

We share these pleasures, giving and receiving.

This is a beloved mind dependent on you for entertainment, stimulation, pleasure, human integrity. In health, we stimulate the minds and imaginations of those we love all the time—remembering to share a funny story or a bit of family news, recommending a book or a website, recalling the past. In awful disability this pleasure continues, perhaps is even enhanced.

There's a satisfaction, even a joy, in getting to the end of a long day with a sense that you've made it. All the many tasks got done, all the trash is out, all the receipts are filed, all the calls were made. Simply surviving a long day of care without getting depressed or anxious is a sort of joy.

Then there is the joyful thanks that this person is still living, still with you, still in this life. It won't always be so, and, however arduous and even tragic, this is better than the alternative.

Hope of recovery—never not there—is another source of joy. Some small percentage of people do recover. Some diseases find new therapies or even a cure. And possibly, just possibly, the terminal-seeming failure of neuromuscular disease or diabetes, dementia or cancer will suddenly be redeemed. AIDS therapies turned a terminal scourge into a chronic, manageable disorder. Leukemia was once a death sentence. To despair of any possible hope is not reasonable. This is not delusional but one piece of your armor against despair.

K

Kindness

Family and faithful friends, former students and caring neighbors, passersby, staff at the dentist's office, the optometrist: the list of people who were more than kind to us over the years is long and wonderful. Pastor colleagues, especially the blessed John Rollefson, who came with communion and good cheer every week, year after year, rain or shine, stand out. And numbers of parishioners remained faithful, sending along art work by their children, bringing the children and food and flowers and friendship.

These people had fine intuition as to what would please and relieve us. They were quick to ask what we might need—which was mostly companionship and good company, those impromptu little parties which nurtured and heartened us.

But two memories are especially remarkable:

The one is of an Indian gentleman in the local park in Los Angeles. When Mariana took Gary to the park on his outings and the Indian man was there, he bowed before Gary in reverence, somehow understanding the special standing of my poor disabled husband as a holy person, set apart and privileged with peace and wisdom. That veneration, across cultures and across religions, was a profound kindness and has stuck with me. So the holy recluses who were shut up in cathedral walls, living cut off in prayer, were honored. So the Trappists choose silence.

The other memory was from a couple of years later. I had made reservations at a big hotel and hauled Gary to Woodland Hills in the chair, in the van, with full life support. When we arrived, I discovered that the bed in our room was on a platform and that it was impossible to lower

Gary onto the bed in the usual manner. Bravely and foolishly, I tipped the lift and sort of dropped him onto the bed with a little crash. I spent a sleepless night worrying how on earth I would get him up off the surface of the bed.

In the morning I asked for a rollaway bed and for any bellhops with any experience in ambulance or hospital work. Three strapping young men appeared a few moments later. We improvised a draw sheet and they transferred my husband effortlessly from the bed to the rollaway. The rest was a breeze—I could take it from there. The lift fit tidily under the rollaway and now we could do the bathing, the dressing and the transfer back to the chair. We would have a great day. The bellhops wouldn't take any money at all—they were very kind—good kids whose parents should be very proud of them.

L

Laptops, iPods, MP3s and the TV

My husband was fond of computers and electronic gadgets. We had a primitive Radio Shack computer back in the early 1980s that used Basic. Then, every year or so for thirty years, we replaced the old machine with a newer model. (Many of the cables are still in the garage.)

So I suppose it was appropriate that every day began for me with a download session. I turned on the laptop and plugged the iPod into the USB drive. While the iPod talked to the computer and shared information, I brewed my morning coffee. Coffee in hand, I returned to sift and filter and arrange my husband's playlist.

The playlist provided many hours of entertainment, intellectual stimulation and music. I had a long page of podcasts that were downloaded whenever a new item was added. So we began with a daily devotion from "Pray as You Go." The *New York Times* podcast followed. Then there were many possibilities, depending on the day of the week. Numbers of National Public Radio shows are podcast. So too American

Public Radio. He caught Garrison Keillor, Slate, How Stuff Works, the *NYT* Science podcast and various sports shows. There were weekly subscriptions to the *New Yorker* and also Zocalo.

My goal was three or four hours daily of fresh news, opinion, entertainment and music. I shaped the list in a familiar sequence. Most of the items were recordings that I would have enjoyed if I had had the time—modified and supplemented with sports and popular science.

Then there were the books. Frankly, Gary was the best-read person I knew. He had three accounts with Audible.com and listened to award-winning fiction and thrillers, politics, biography, history—and a round of Bible texts. When an author showed up on the Daily Show, Gary had almost always read the book. I skimmed book reviews and best-seller lists and shopped for bargains on classics. His "library" on Audible.com was immense.

Nor did I despise TV. Given the limited number of hours he could watch TV (his eyes dried out as he could not blink and tending them with ointments and saline drops was pretty strenuous), I used the DVR and planned ahead. I recorded what I could to watch later—including, always, the Daily Show and the Colbert Report, Bill Maher and Meet the Press. While not a sports fan myself, I tracked the playoffs and anything NBA or NFL. I even tried to keep tabs on college basketball and football in their seasons. Some standard crime shows are rich in dialogue (Law and Order, Criminal Minds). These could be mostly listened to without eyestrain. Other shows required that I close Gary's eyes during the commercials.

I promised myself that boredom would not be the death of my clever husband and, if anything, erred on the side of overstimulation.

I tried the computerized reading of books and magazines on the Kindle. (I suppose I could have tried harder.) Friends recorded some texts on CDs and I converted those files to MP3s.

Volume was a constant issue as different podcasts and other recordings seemed to be too loud or too soft and both I and my caregivers needed to stay alert to sound levels.

I suspect that my morning routine of loading the iPod was the most valuable thing I did as a caregiver. It was a pleasure to manage his day's entertainment and then to be able to move on to my own affairs.

The laptop was also a crucial means of training and retaining caregivers. They took notes and kept timesheets on the computer. They were welcome to use it for homework, email, shopping or other personal purposes. (It had very fine security software.)

Living Richly

One of my promises to myself was that Gary would never die of neglect. The other was that I would provide the richest possible life for him that I could arrange. Doing so meant drawing on all the experience of all our years together.

After he was tracheostomized and attached to a ventilator, he almost entirely lost all sense of smell. (Sometimes, he spelled, when he was being turned, he would catch a bit of a scent.) When he could no longer swallow safely he could only eat passively, through the stomach tube.

Gary had always delighted in good food, in good coffee, in the scents of the out-of-doors and in the scents of flowers and perfumes. He had always selected perfumes for me and for our daughters, and we trusted his good nose and his good judgment.

I always ate my dinner at his side. When the family came to visit, they too ate with him—or we carted him in to sit near the family table. I trusted, indeed I believe, that the olfactory memory is the strongest, most basic memory. I, certainly, with a much lesser sense of smell, can imagine smells when I read recipes or look at a picture of a scrumptious meal. The delight is real. He must have shared in the pleasure of flavors and scents remembered as he shared our company.

Somewhere I read an opinion that it was mean to eat in front of somebody who can't. I disagree.

Physical intimacy is also such a mix of memory and desire that the different sort of sexual relations we enjoy with a terribly disabled life partner are much like food. Just as the brain remembers the smell of a slice of good pizza or the taste of a great margarita, so the body remembers touch and arousal and the pleasures of intercourse. Whatever we can or can no longer do in bed, it's all connected to what we have known in the past. If the hands that once stroked me passionately could no longer move, when I placed them on my body and moved beneath them, the memory—for both of us, I assumed—did the rest.

Food and sex, the senses and the memory, are foundational to any marriage. We were around sixty when our particular disaster struck, but younger couples in a similar situation have successfully conceived children.

The richness I sought was also one of mutual pleasure in comedy and tragedy, in music and books and the beach, in family time and friendly visits. I also tried to honor the richness of Gary's life that I didn't especially share—especially the sports (NBA, NFL and collegiate athletics). I learned how to find the games I knew he would love and to make certain he caught them. I was always careful to include thrillers and biography in his playlists so that there was Tom Clancy as well as Jeffrey Eugenides.

Early in our saga, more than ten years ago, soon after Gary was silenced by the tracheostomy and when he had just invented the communication system, spooked by the doctors, I was sure he was dying. He spelled out "f" "i" "n" "a" "l"—and my heart went to my throat, sure he was going to make some final request. Then came the next letters "f" "o" "u" "r". He wanted to make really sure he didn't miss the Final Four of the NCAA basketball season.

M

"Moving On" (for church people)

Three times in as many years friends suggested that the church Gary served when he became ill needed to "move on." They have said this to explain the lack of attention from the church people, their failure (after an initial flurry) to visit or call, their total indifference to our acute need for friendship and compassion. The expression "to move on" puzzled me. It hurt deeply.

I've done some research and it seems the expression is pretty exclusively used to describe failed relationships, divorces and the like. A very odd model for the church's relationship to its stricken pastor! Was Gary's paralysis perceived as infidelity? He cheated the church by becoming ill and so the church had to "move on" for its own well-being?

In the parable of the Good Samaritan, the priest and the Pharisee "pass by on the other side." They don't exactly "move on." They never had nor have they sought a neighborly relationship with the man who fell among thieves and lay, half dead, by the road. That reaction seems, rather, to describe the bishops and other church authorities who failed to help Gary or me in our situation. According to the parable, they are in bad spiritual trouble of their own! (Indeed, the ELCA church hierarchy—as it seized Gary's Social Security through the process of "offsetting" his benefits, then stripped him of his disability benefits altogether, then took away his health insurance—may more resemble the thieves than the passersby.)

The parable doesn't explain the members of his church. I suspect that their model is rather the goofy model of a pastor as spouse of the congregation who somehow failed his people by getting sick so that they, like a long-suffering wife, must "move on" from the failed relationship. That is utterly sick, depraved and perverse, but who ever said that congregations have healthy relationships with their "beloved" pastors?

The three friends who justified the abandonment in the language of the congregation "moving on" were all respectable church people—one a pastor, two lay leaders. All three were in faithful, long-term personal relationships. Somehow they all picked up on the same odd language of the culture of divorce. They may have meant to comfort me. In fact, their comfort was very cold, much colder than the comfort offered Job by his friends.

My Generation of (Women) Caregivers

My generation—we who were young women in the early seventies—felt we were the first to tackle motherhood alongside professional lives. We had no sense that we were simply part of the collapse of the economic structures that had given men a generous enough wage so the little woman could reproduce and keep house without too much stress. Such cynicism was far from our thoughts as we bravely exhausted ourselves.

So I took my doctoral exams within a few months of giving birth ("naturally" of course) to our first child. I wrote my dissertation while nursing a newborn (literally) and trudged to the typist pushing a stroller with the second infant in a Snugli. (A total novelty in Manhattan in 1973, you could only find one through the *Whole Earth Catalog*.) I discovered I was pregnant with our third daughter while working on a book in London and she was born before I quite had tenure. Three small children, a book, tenure and, all the while, intensive involvement with church work as my husband was a pastor and I always took the role of pastor's spouse pretty seriously.

Changing diapers, tending sick children, cooking and baking were complements to the heady work of writing, lecturing, grading and editing. There were innumerable joys and pleasures to lighten the hard work and the late nights. I also hired help. Babysitters and housecleaners were as familiar in my household as they had been in the home in which I grew up. And my husband was very good at carrying his share of the load. That was the standard. And he had grown up in a farm family in which gender was less important than getting a job done. So we worked side by side.

It occurs to me that my generation may also be the first seriously to combine home care of invalids with professional endeavors. My kids never were put in daycare. So my beloved husband would never be installed in a "facility." I managed their feces and urine and vomit and comforted them without neglecting my scholarly obligations. Just so I lectured and graded and wrote and edited this and that between the duties of emptying the cath bag, administering enemas and crushing pills to dissolve in liquid to inject into the g-tube. Always and forever, day and night, were the back-numbing turns, side-to-side, and the perfect positioning of my husband's inert, heavy, 6'4" frame.

I was not alone. I may be on the leading edge, but professional women caring for invalid husbands will certainly proliferate over the next decades. And of course nearly as many men care for their spouses tenderly and joyfully. Cutting edge? Perhaps—but certainly less obviously an adventure.

I suspect that caring for elderly and dependent parents is a different issue. The load may be shared with siblings and even children. There were years of planning and preparation, perhaps a gradual decline into senescence.

Husbands or wives or partners stricken by disease in their prime are another, stranger story. Surely both the sense of romance and the sense of tragedy are stronger.

Modern Medicine

Modern medicine, especially neurology, has simply failed us. Like those caring for loved ones suffering from the awful list that includes Parkinson's, Alzheimer's, MS and ALS, I followed the breaking news of this or that study or clinical trial—in the few minutes I could spare from hands-on care or the supervision of the caregivers I hired to help in this arduous business of long-term care.

Regularly, people asked me questions about my husband's condition, wanting details and diagnosis. I shared what I could, but also explained that his "diagnosis" was purely descriptive (Chronic Inflammatory, Demyelinating Polyneuropathy), that there was no cure, that there was really no prognosis, so let's, please, not dwell on the science?

Doctors are trained to drive for diagnosis, to drive for the fix or else put you in the hands of the mild and understanding "Palliative Medicine" crew with their hospice care and pain management—not a bad thing under certain circumstances, but by no means useful for those of us dealing with chronic, mysterious disability. The few humble doctors who seem to get it, to continue care, to leave room for miracles, to honor their patients and their patients' families' choices, are more precious than rubies.

Friends have introduced, almost as offerings, a raft of interesting alternative medical solutions. So, early on, a "healer" from the mountains of Southern California was brought to our home by earnest friends. She was something of a witch, SoCal style, with brightly colored, blowsy clothing and a mass of frizzy hair. She used touch and some sort of rituals. (I seem to recall that I stepped outside, overcome with the giggles!) A parishioner felt her Sikh chiropractor was the solution and for many months he and his assistant cracked my husband's neck, prescribed sessions on a foot vibration device, invented that great trapeze and recommended various herbal preparations. Another earnest, pale young man named Duane visited several times. He wept in pity, did a bit of acupuncture and put us on his email list. He surfaces in my inbox every couple of months, providing tips on natural living. Then there was a Christian healing service that included lots and lots of oil. The oil dripped into my husband's eyes, which became very red and stung madly.

More scientific, if experimental, treatments were no more successful and included costly human growth hormone injections and intravenous immune globulin therapy.

A neighbor with awful, deep-brain Parkinson's has been to China for stem cell therapy. Mexican clinics have always drawn US citizens desperate for help. And a memory comes back to me from my childhood how doctor relatives in Germany specialized in a process whereby the cells of freshly slaughtered calf liver were injected into rich pilgrims from South America who wanted a new lease on life. I do not mean to denigrate any of these quests or any of these healing practices. I understand the impulse to look for unconventional solutions very well and I resist.

N

Neglect

One of my promises to myself and to Gary was that he would never die of neglect—not personal neglect, not professional neglect. The personal promise was easier to keep than the professional. I loved him and loved being close. The care of his body was second nature to me. The care of his mind was a joy.

The possibility of physical neglect lurked everywhere. Chilling or overheating were always dangers because California indoor temperatures can range from the high fifties to the upper nineties. Besides the furnace and the air conditioner my resources included a drawer of socks, a heating pad, a space heater and a fan, and a selection of blankets ranging from very light to very warm.

Just so, hydration in the summer was really important, so I studied the color of his urine like some doctor of the distant past and adjusted the quantity of water we poured into his feeding tube accordingly.

His skin was prone to breakdown, which meant constant observation and another drawer of ointments and powders, creams and patches (duoderm, tegaderm).

His eyes needed lubrication and careful rinsing. His fingertips needed to be soaked and then pushed carefully back from the nail or they would bleed when trimmed. (The skin adhered to the nail because his fingers were unused.)

His ears and neck could grow fungus if they were damp. His "stomae," the holes in his neck and stomach and abdomen, needed to be clean and dry.

But I have known people who take better care of their dogs!

O

OTC—Over-the-Counter Supplies

This is a very shaky category. It sounds like the stock of things one buys at the drugstore—gauze and hydrogen peroxide, antiseptic wipes and liquid Tylenol, applicator swabs (Q-Tips) and alcohol pads. But in fact, some of these things are paid for by insurance—and so come from your home care supplier—some are not. And what gets paid by insurance seems to change randomly. So gauze pads and applicator swabs were not supplied by insurance in Los Angeles but in San Diego they came in a big box from Apria.

What's more, the local drugstore chain (with its "counter") is likely not competitive with online suppliers. Perhaps careful shopping would uncover local stores with deals, but that kind of shopping takes time, time that is suddenly worth the $15-$20 per hour paid to a caregiver plus the gas money.

Sometimes visiting nurses will supply a goodly number of exam gloves. Sometimes not.

Many items not requiring a prescription may be covered by insurance but you never quite know which.

Supplying a home hospital is really complicated. Different caregivers have different expectations and what is de rigueur for one nurse is useless to another.

Here's a basic list:

Exam gloves in the right size. (They come small, medium, large in boxes of 100. Some are latex, some vinyl. Some are pre-powdered, some not.) Because they are taught to change gloves every few minutes, helpers who have worked in a "facility" can go through a whole box in twelve hours. I tried to moderate this excess, but didn't want to be cheap.

These can cost a small fortune at the drug store but are available for pennies through an online source like Allegro Medical or even Amazon. Order a thousand medium in vinyl, not powdered, to start.

Disposable underpads, commonly known as "chux." These come in various sizes and various degrees of absorbency. The smaller and less absorbent the less they cost. An incontinent patient may go through many in the course of a day. A catheterized (tube in the bladder) patient uses far fewer. Like gloves, they are best ordered in bulk. They save laundry, soak up spills and work well for training puppies and changing babies. (Washable underpads also have their uses and may be more environmentally friendly.)

Washcloths. Buy these in bulk from Costco or Amazon or Overstock.com. They get stained, they wear out, they are nasty before you know it. Twenty is not too many for a single invalid. You may find yourself using them to bring down a fever.

Towels. I prefer good quality but not too thick, bleachable white so any stains are evident. Try shopping online.

Toiletries include Aveeno Body Wash, lotion and Vaseline. I stuck with my husband's favorite shampoo, scent and deodorant and found it important that he smelled familiar. The idea of buying fine perfume for somebody immobilized and unable to communicate may seem like a silly extravagance, but I found it an essential part of preserving his identity. I assume that dementia patients and the comatose are similarly well served by smelling like themselves to their loved ones.

OTC medicines in our stash included multivitamin tablets, Vitamin C, acidophilus capsules, baby aspirin, cranberry extract.

You can save money on many of these supplies through Amazon.com, particularly their Prime membership where shipping is paid in a lump sum. I had regular deliveries of shampoo, vitamins, suppositories, enemas and baby wipes from Amazon through their "Subscribe and Save" program.

Supermarket supplies include distilled vinegar (mixed 1:4 with water for disinfection), bleach, laundry detergent and prune juice.

Order

My first principle of domestic order in our little private hospital was that equipment and supplies, medicines and even staff back braces all be hidden from view. The utter junkiness of the alternative is very distressing. We lived in a home, not a hospital, and homes are gracious and tidy spaces.

Our beds were "adjustable" beds that I slid together in the evening—so I could sleep with my hand under Gary's after I had positioned him for the night. During the day, his bed was accessible from all four sides for various nursing tasks. At night a boudoir, in the day an ICU!

This was hard to communicate to the people I paid to help. Their training and experience had often been in clinical situations. They weren't especially sympathetic to the idea of my home. (They weren't bothered by urological supplies left out in plain sight.)

I have often thought that my model was less like an ICU and more like a modern birthing suite where all the medicines and high-tech equipment are hidden from view. Like birth, home care is natural and comforting, a place for family and the enjoyment of one another. Signs of anything else are distracting.

My second principle was that all the gear and supplies, from boxes of saline ampules to vent filters and suppositories, from extra tubing to blood pressure cuffs—all of it must have a logical place where it was easy to find. This, too, took a great deal of effort. Mariana (see "Saints' Choir," below) moved us into our home in the middle of a semester. It took me months after she left to sort and order our supplies to my satisfaction—and Mariana was a hospital-trained nurse. The system must be obvious to anybody.

My third principle was that items used many times a day were within ten feet of Gary's bed—mostly in bedside drawers. Items used once or twice a day were in baskets, labeled "grooming," "trach care," "bowel bin," and put back properly on their shelves after use. These were to be stocked regularly so there was no sudden shortage.

Labels and cardstock lists and printed instructions all help with such order. It's well worth the time it takes to set up the system and to tweak it as necessary. The more sense it makes, the easier to communicate the system to your people.

Caregivers who jumble baskets and bins and who fail to report shortages are really not doing what they are paid to do.

P

Plan of Care

A "plan of care" is a technical term, used by nurses, to describe everything entailed in a day of nursing care. It's in nursing code and leaves out lots of tasks (like emptying a catheter bag or washing a load of towels) that a nurse just takes for granted.

My own plans of care were more like blow-by-blow duties, written out for a reminder or for a newbie. I asked caregivers who had worked with us for a spell to write down everything they did in a shift (using the staff laptop). Then I could keep up to date—or eliminate tasks that were no longer necessary.

Such a highly detailed list of tasks is a good management tool. It also helps when a caregiver goes on vacation or quits or simply doesn't show up to work. It helped me measure the quality of work and reminded me just how much my helpers did.

I have placed a daily plan of care in the Appendix at the end of this book. It might serve as a model or just help you make sense of one fairly extreme situation.

Political Reflections

I have personally saved the government several millions on health care. My motives were ethical and romantic rather than patriotic and those were hard years, but there were many gratifications and even joy. I learned a great deal about human nature and medicine and love. I don't know to what extent my model is replicable, but I guess it's time to share:

I was 64 and the primary caregiver—in our home—for a husband who was 67 when he died and so acutely disabled that, when he did go to the hospital, only the Intensive Care Unit (ICU) had the equipment and the personnel to manage his care. My husband was totally paralyzed, speechless, unable to open his eyes without the help of a headband I devised. My husband breathed via ventilator, ate canned liquid through a stomach tube, and peed through another tube in his poor abdomen. (The management of his bowels was another story.)

He had to be turned from one side to the other every hour, carefully repositioned with pillows with every turn to manage pressure sores. He had to be bathed and groomed daily. Because he remained mentally and emotionally himself (we had to assume), I provided a steady stream of good reading (books, magazines, lectures, newspapers) via IPod. He stayed current on a range of sports and politics. He watched favorite TV shows. His children and grandchildren visited regularly. He received weekly visits from his pastor and occasional visits from friends.

I slept next to him every night, rising to suction his trachea when the alarm on the ventilator sounded. During the day, when I showered, I turned off the water every thirty seconds or so to listen for the alarm.

When he was well (no sores or respiratory problems) and I had help, we went outside. This involved a sling, an electronic lift, a complex transfer protocol, the huge wheelchair with a shelf for the ventilator, and great care. Sometimes we used the van to go to church or to a daughter's house.

When we went to the hospital, he was uncomfortable, he contracted infections, he was not regularly bathed or turned. They couldn't believe I cared for him at home. One day in the ICU cost tens of thousands of dollars. One day at home cost the government very, very little (just vent rental and miscellaneous supplies).

I hired help using money from family donations and from my work teaching. But the help needed extensive training and the helpers tended to burn out fast, despite all my positive reinforcement and support. It was a struggle.

I know I am not the only caregiver in the United States. We are legion. I know that my situation was not nearly as dire as that of people of lesser means with less support caring for profoundly disabled family members. We all simply love whom we love and do what we can.

As a Baby Boomer and a feminist, I am a long-time observer of the choices facing working moms, the unpleasant arguments of who is better and what is best. I am a great believer in choice in these matters, considered and careful choice. Just so, in my situation, I could not help but wonder just how much nursing home care and acute hospital care and even government or private insurance-managed home care could be replaced by safer, more economical home care. I suspect that a compassionate, supportive system is possible and would be transformative.

The analogy here is with a parent making a modest salary who must put her kids in daycare to work, daycare that costs everything the parent is earning. What if the parent would rather be with her kids, providing a better standard of care than the daycare offers? What if all she needs is some modest financial support, some respite care and positive reinforcement?

Why does our system provide healthcare and benefits for a batty mother of 14 children (conceived in vitro) and leave us without help?

A word about licensed vocational nurses (LVNs): For the first 18 months or so of our trial, we had good insurance that provided 70 hours a week of in-home nursing care. The insurance benefit was, however, much better than the nurses. The agency received, from the insurance, something like $35 per hour for nurses who got, with luck, $20.00 and some funky benefits. A couple of the nurses were competent. Others lied about their hours, cheated, or spent all the time on cell phones or watching TV. They would prop my husband in front of daytime TV, stark naked, and criticize everything about my management of my household and his care. Clearly that's not a healthcare system but a scam.

I am not a policy wonk, a journalist, or a public health specialist. I could have, I suppose, if I had had a moment to spare (which I didn't), looked some of these things up. But I suspect the statistics are profoundly confusing and depend (as always) on the agenda of the researcher. I'm sure that the vested interests, including home health agencies, professional social workers, hospitals and the many nursing homes and care facilities out there are all opposed to the profound revision I am imagining.

One of the many challenges is that home caregivers are lonely and isolated, deprived of the social network that's the norm in the workplace. Something like the nannies in the local park who talk nonstop on their cellphones, the profession attracts unskilled people without the resources to be alone. These problems can all be solved and many billions saved over the coming years.

Pressure Sores

Bed sores, pressure sores, pressure ulcers, skin breakdown, excoriation—the language used to describe what happens to the skin of a bed-bound patient is rich and descriptive. The skin cannot take the constant, immobile weight of the body and it collapses. It breaks down in a series of terrible stages. Sores from sitting immobile in a wheelchair are no nicer than the ones from lying immobile in a bed, so "pressure sore" is a better term.

In my experience, hospital nurses are better at photo-documenting pressure sores and giving them a "stage" number than they are at healing them. For example, hospital protocol calls for "turning" patients from one position to another (left side, back, right side) every two hours. The second hour is excruciatingly painful for the immobile quadriplegic, but that doesn't seem to matter to nurses. Nor does the "team" required to turn ever show up on time. So without advocacy and intervention, the intervals stretch to three and even four hours.

At home, turns can be managed much better. I turned my husband every hour—the interval he had requested when he could communicate. In fact, his blood pressure—the indicator of his pain—rose in the ten minutes before a turn. It came down again as soon as he was properly positioned.

Other factors that affect the development of pressure sores include protein consumption, something I learned way too late in the game. For somebody fed by tube, getting sufficient protein powder is an essential component of good care.

Q

Quantities and Inventory

One of our many challenges was to assure that there was plenty of everything we needed on hand but not such an oversupply that the cupboards and drawers were overflowing.

As with maintaining order, controlling inventory can be a challenge to teach.

In the early days it would drive me crazy when a nurse would suddenly declare that we were out of shampoo or out of chux or out of gloves. I had to stop whatever I was doing and run to the store to buy a supply, usually at ruinous expense.

I discovered that simply watching inventory was a high-order skill that didn't belong to the skill set of home care nurses. I took to asking "is there anything we need?" several times a week. And whenever I was on my own, with no help, as happened occasionally, I used a chunk of the downtime for basic inventory.

As disturbing, perhaps, was the sort of hoarding that many helpers practiced. No quantity was ever too much and I'd discover that we had three years' worth of vent circuits or trach ties, none of which could be returned.

R

Care providers, the bad and the good, become a huge part of the lives of caregivers and their patients. Who they are and where they come from, their apparent motives and practices, all become central features of your daily life in a care situation. I have divided profiles of some of the more notable caregivers into two categories—the rogues and the saints. (All names have been changed.)

Rogues' Gallery:

Patsy

Patsy was only in our lives for a couple of months. She looked like a really sweet person in her caregiver profile on Care.com—blonde, perky, wearing a stylish cap. She had a college degree, something to do with computers, and an interest in helping out while she built her business in web design. She showed up on time and sank into the couch, all three hundred pounds of her. I worried about her health and her stamina as well as my chairs, but found that if she rested regularly she did well. I was concerned about her back, but the brace I provide for nursing staff didn't fit her girth. She said her back was strong, that she could bend to the floor, just like her large grandmother.

She had had bariatric surgery. She had had foot surgery. I heard her tell a coworker that she had adult onset muscular dystrophy, a genetic condition. She didn't tolerate water on her skin and couldn't wash tubing or suction canisters. She had a latex allergy and needed vinyl gloves.

Nobody's perfect, but Patsy clearly had issues. She kept dogs and spoke to Gary as though he were a large dog. Never married and childless, she talked fondly about her nieces and nephews. She talked a lot.

I encouraged caregivers to read, work online, to make personal use of the hours of downtime that went with caring for Gary. Patsy wanted to work—and proceeded to manage the supplies and the linens with amazing skill. Never have I seen washcloths rolled into such tight cylinders and towels and sheets and shirts folded so very, very flat. She tended to tell me what to do, but I didn't especially mind. She also tended to tell other people on the staff what to do and to impugn their orderliness.

Then, suddenly, everything went very, very wrong. She wanted to talk. My sweet housecleaner was leaving for the day shortly, so I told Patsy we'd talk after she left. I had a nice chat with the housecleaner. Patsy pushed for her time. I asked how much time she needed. She said about fifteen minutes. When I made the time, she launched into a tirade about how it was all about me and my needs, what about her? (In fact I paid her well to help me with my needs. This was not a relationship of mutual needs.) I really think she was jealous of my talking with the housecleaner! I said I counted on her time on duty to get my own work done. She blew up and quit—on the spot—demanding her check. I said I would need a timesheet. She stormed out of the house, returned half an hour later with her time sheet, across which she had scrawled "I quit," took her check and left.

Sissy

This all happened about a month after Sissy, another helper, went to prison. She had been helping with the house and with Gary on the days when I had no nursing support. We had found one another on Craigslist three months earlier. I knew she lived close to the edge, but her cleaning energies were astonishing and she had passed my informal drug test—an old bottle of Vicodin in the medicine cabinet upstairs. A family crisis had rendered her homeless at Christmastime and I had taken her in for a couple of nights, until she found another place to stay. (She wasn't all there, but who really is? And her energies, even if drug-enhanced, were a marvel.)

When the DEA agent called to ask if the check in her purse was indeed her check from me, I was puzzled. He had picked her up on an outstanding warrant. A neighbor who used to work for the Public Defender showed me how to trace her progress through the criminal justice system. Felony grand theft. She never cashed her check. She was released a couple of months later and I took her back for help on weekends. She was very nice, a hard worker, and I trusted her (within limits). I also was desperate on weekends.

Simba

When Sissy stayed with us for those two nights Simba was still in the house. Simba, also a Craigslist find, was my introduction to the category of "senior caregiver." She had spent years moving from one home of one elderly person needing companionship to another. Never certified or trained, she specialized in kindness and low-grade service. She claimed to have had really bad experiences with Christians and to now be a Buddhist. I rose to the bait.

She thought she could learn the intricacies of Gary's care but never really managed. She was inappropriately self-confident, which was really dangerous in our situation. I suspect she had a serious learning disability. She couldn't handle money or make very clear judgments about life goals. Unable or unwilling to drive, she travelled far and wide by bus, a real challenge in north San Diego County. I don't think she ever really knew where she was, geographically or metaphorically. For Christmas I gave her a nice jacket. Our gathered family suspected something was wrong when she couldn't figure out the zipper. We worried that somebody who couldn't manage a zipper would not do well managing the intricacies of life support.

Initially, on the phone interview, she had said she wanted to go back to college and major in anthropology. She had also been told she had a good voice and was interested in radio broadcasting. She had very few belongings and traveled light. She got really hungry every couple of hours and helped herself until I explained that room, not board, was what I had offered. Thereafter she asked me to pick up fried chicken whenever I went to the store.

I thought we had arranged for her to work in exchange for her room and bath plus a good stipend. She understood that she'd have a free room and a generous salary. She had been paying $600 per month for a room before she moved in with us. I offered her a $500 deal. When she got her first check she burst into tears! She stayed for another miserable month, exerting herself minimally, winding through the landscape on one bus after another, finally leaving for her new job with a healthy check in hand.

Bork
As it became clear that Simba would not work out, I had contacted Bork, who had formerly worked for us and was on his third "time out." I called these his time outs, these periods of a month or two when we had fought and he was no longer working in our house. I wanted to know if Bork

wanted to come back—on clear terms—no dependence on his mother for transportation; no arguing with me about matters of fact; reasonable respect and communication. He never responded.

At that point Bork had worked for us off and on for most of a year. Sickly with some horrible stomach disorder, like Sissy he was heavily tattooed. (His knuckles bore the inscription B O R N F R E E, which was very far from his particular reality.) When he first came into our lives he had lost his driver's license for speeding. He got it back several months later and, using money he had earned working for us and in a "facility," bought a car—an ancient sports car, a 40-year-old Datsun. He drove it to work a couple of times and then the mechanical difficulties began. He rarely came to work because he had to "work on his car" with a friend who could only help on weekends, the days I especially needed help. Then he lost his job at the care facility—for sleeping on his shift, the night shift. We lost touch for a spell there, then he was back.

He had decided he wanted to study martial arts and asked whether I knew anybody in China. He confessed to a houseguest from the Middle East that he was the heir to the Ottoman Empire—according to his Turkish father. Meanwhile, he could only work when his mother was able to bring him to our house and then to pick him up. She spent as many hours on the road, bringing him back and forth, as he spent actually on the job. When his nursing duties were done, he shopped for car parts online.

He was very willing to help with odd jobs around the house although tended to dent and chip walls and furniture and generally run into things and needed continuous supervision. His acute fear of spiders limited his usefulness in the garage but he did a good job washing the car.

Once I loaned him my car, giving very clear instructions to only drive it between my house and his house. I googled the mileage and checked the odometer. He added in around 50 miles that day and claimed that the freeway was congested and he'd had to take surface roads. I put him on time out.

(Cars)

Cars are a big issue with the people who work in home care. The costs of owning a car and driving a car never seem to compute and applicants from faraway communities apply for jobs with little sense of the expense involved. When I challenged them—on the phone or in person—they were sure it wasn't a problem. Then, over time, the truth would come clear. When you're making $12 or $15/hour you cannot afford to drive 100 miles round trip for a 6-hour shift. And the cars tend to be old and in a state of disrepair. Very possibly the odometer is a mystery and mpg so much technobabble.

I was not unsympathetic. I believe people can learn, can learn lifelong. I think I am a good and patient teacher. Perhaps I was too patient and expected to help my workers get a better grip on life while they worked with us. Perhaps I was too willing to believe the impressive self-presentation of applicants primed for job interviews.

After writing this, I again heard from Bork. He thought I should loan him $600 to pay the mechanic for car repairs and to pay the DMV for the registration. He would work the debt off however and whenever I needed help—but not that particular, upcoming weekend. I had to say no.

Matt

When we lived in Los Angeles, during the first eighteen months of Gary's paralysis, before the church dumped him onto Medicare (for the neurologically diseased), we received seventy hours of paid help per week, this was arranged through an agency. That was where we first encountered the rogues who staff home health agencies. Like the people I have hired in recent years, using Craigslist and Care.com, these nurses (technically LVNs who are vent-certified) live very close to the edge. They tend to have elaborate fantasies about what life holds in store for them.

Matt had trained as a nurse in the army. Now he was in college and in a band. He was a really personable kid and encouraged us to get out and go places. (He had worked for a man with ALS and had good practical sense. He had worked as an EMT and managed the wheelchair in the van nicely.) Perhaps the band and the girlfriend explained why he was as many as six hours late most days. He would show up at one or two in the afternoon when he was due at eight in the morning. I called and called. Then he would want to stay until nine or ten at night—which was not OK with me.

Matt regularly had me sign his paperwork before he had filled it out. I was too naïve to suspect that I was in fact a party to major insurance fraud.

Finally, when I complained to the agency that I wasn't getting my 10-hour days from Matt, they disputed my claim. He had logged ten hours on all those five- and six-hour days. He was nothing more than a charming crook who had defrauded me and my husband, the agency and the insurance company.

James
Perhaps most bizarre—and sad, I suppose—are the fantasy worlds so many caregivers seem to inhabit. One middle-aged man, an agency nurse who worked for us for many months, told stories about how he had formerly been in finance, the field in which he earned his university degree back in Guam—or was it the Philippines? (He changed his island of origin when I introduced him to a friend from Guam.) When we took Gary to a movie in the Century City mall where lots of business people from the surrounding office buildings go for lunch, he recalled his days in a fancy suit and tie. Such stories combined strangely with his account of his elderly parents and the disabled siblings who were dependent upon him.

Soon after the agency sent him to work for us he had asked for a loan, something like $1,200. He needed help for his family. This is, of course, a total no-no. When caregivers ask clients for money awful scenarios of abuse loom, particularly for clients less alert and cautious than I. I explained that this was unethical and, however sympathetic, I couldn't possibly cross that line.

Several weeks later he remarked about our big-screen plasma TV that he had a number of such at his house. I said, "but James, how could you afford so many?" He said he'd bought them several years ago. I observed that they had cost many thousands of dollars even then. He changed the subject.

Like many of his colleagues, James's skills as a nurse varied from day to day. In public he was prone to removing a key filter piece in the ventilator line and shaking out the condensation. As I explained to him many times, the whole point of that filter was to hydrate the air in the vent, but that wasn't my main complaint. The removal risked introducing microbes of various kinds into Gary's lungs! James refused to defer to my arguments and I could no longer risk adventures away from home. Just so, his version of the "bowel program" involved rhythmic (disturbingly suggestive, actually) manual probing. I finally asked that he not be sent again when I came home to find my husband, stark naked, propped upright in bed—no glasses, no headphones. James explained that he was watching TV.

S

Saints' Choir

Even the best caregivers burn out, turning critical or sullen or losing their focus. The loneliness of the work and the long hours take their toll. When the course of a disease is endless, unremitting and incurable it is hard to remain sharp and devoted, whatever the pay, whatever the perquisites. To celebrate the good nurses and caregivers I have had to rewind my memory to the months before things got ugly, to the good times.

Raymond
We lured Raymond from the facility.

After Gary flunked out of the rehab program and we understood that we couldn't move back to our walk-up apartment, we landed in a "board and care," run by what I can only describe as two crazy Romanians. The wife said she had been a doctor in her homeland but was an RN in the US. The husband had been a dentist in Romania but was now just an opinionated chain smoker. They had acquired two large properties and turned them into "board and care" residential facilities. The one we moved into was almost empty, which may have been why I was allowed to live there too, which was the whole idea. I needed to learn to care for Gary, to find a way.

Raymond was one of two caregivers at the facility. Both were Filipino. Raymond, he said, had come to the US on a work visa, recruited to work in DC (so he had a social security number). The work was oppressive and he had left, taking the bus to California, where he found work as a caregiver. He was strong and gentle, knowledgeable and kind. He worked at the home 24/7 for a very low wage with occasional days off when he would return to the home very red-eyed, very hung over. We would eventually learn that he also had a serious gambling addiction, a wife and two daughters in the Philippines, and a love of cars. He would rather be a cook than a caregiver and would later try his hand in a restaurant.

Raymond moved with us to the downstairs of the duplex in Beverly Hills that would be our home for almost four years. He literally moved us in. He was perfectly reliable, perfectly kind. Ignorant about the gambling, I encouraged him to take other work on the side and to save up. The marriage didn't last. His daughters sent pretty little letters on flowered stationary. I don't know if he even read them.

The other caregiver at the facility had been freed from domestic slavery in Los Angeles. Enslaved by a fellow Filipina, she had shared her story with a casual acquaintance who had reported the situation to the police. The upshot was a visa for her husband, a former teacher, who came to Los Angeles and tried to work in the facility. He was just awful at everything he tried.

I would hear more stories about these terrible separations, wives at home in the Philippines while husbands worked in the US and husbands raising the kids in the islands while the wives worked jobs in LA or Dubai or wherever. The caregivers all have stories, but Raymond's was one of the saddest.

Raymond stayed with us until we found that our insurance would pay for seventy hours of nursing per week. We stayed in touch and he returned later, between other jobs, to help out when the church cancelled our insurance.

Diana
Diana was a real gem—and also, of course, as a lifelong caregiver, something of a piece of work. Sent by the agency, and probably having been told that I was a professor, she showed up with a novel in her bag—by a Chicana writer, no less. (That was the last time in the eighteen months we knew her that I ever saw her even pretend to read anything.)

In keeping with her kind, she harbored grand ambitions. She would go back to school and become a wound care specialist. I wanted to help and looked for programs. Nothing came of that and she even said at one point that she had never been able to think very clearly since the anesthesia they'd given her with her fourth childbirth. When I last saw her she had gone to Mexico and had all her teeth replaced with large, new, very white implants.

I don't know how much of Diana's life story was composed for my entertainment, but it was a doozy. She had been married to an abusive man and produced four children with various drug and crime problems. They had belonged to a radical Christian cult that required them to sever all contact with extended family and destroy photos and mementos. After divorcing him, she had married a younger guy recovering from drug abuse. (I met the younger ex-husband when he visited—after Diana had moved in with us.)

All of Diana's large extended family, their spouses and their in-laws had elaborate stories that she shared with relish. The girlfriend of one son kept "popping babies," their relationship to Diana's son uncertain. Neglected and unsupervised, their teeth were rotten and they were underweight. (I met the two sons who were in trouble with the law, scary guys you wouldn't want to meet on the street late at night. After Diana left us to live with her kids she reported that they lost the apartment after a major brawl.)

Diana was diabetic and very careful with her diet. She was precise in almost everything and took good care of Gary's body—to the extreme point of trimming Gary's body hair for her version of hygienic purposes.

She was also good at the spelling system and communicated effectively and efficiently with Gary, which I took as a sign of her basic intelligence and concern.

She had come to Los Angeles to help care for her aged mother. She left to accompany her son and his family back to Texas, where they lived in a resold FEMA trailer. She held a job at a school for a year or so. By the time she returned to Los Angeles, we had moved to San Diego.

Lindsey
Lindsey responded to an ad I placed on Craigslist—back when Craigslist was still pretty safe. After Diana left I had an extra room with bath, a hot commodity in West LA, and I advertised for somebody who would help with Gary in exchange for a place to live.

She said she had recently graduated from UCLA in Art History—although nothing in her demeanor or among her belongings confirmed that. She had had a dream about a tall woman with white hair before we met and felt that augured good things about me. She moved in committing to ten hours a week of help with Gary and I helped her get a job in a local dress shop.

Her plan was to launch a career as a film producer using a set of strange ideas that never made sense to me and important connections she had made during internships while at UCLA. As the weeks passed she grew whisper thin, dressing in high chic clothing and living on lettuce. When our main caregiver left, I asked if she wanted to work more hours and quit the shop and she agreed to do so.

Lindsey came from an abusive Korean-American background and didn't want her family to know where she was. She had never learned to drive a car. A nasty brother kept calling and calling and reduced her to tears. She told horror stories of the plastic surgery of her friends and family who had their eyelids and their calves altered to Caucasian standards. She was some sort of radical evangelical Christian and spoke in extravagant terms about the wonderful community of church people who loved her so much.

She was a devout virgin who would never marry a Korean. She never dated and had no social life that I could tell. She was big on Hollywood networking—or so it seemed—and the kind of enthusiastic idea vetting that belongs to that world.

She was reasonably attentive and precise. She was clever and a quick study. She was, for the most part, respectful and kind, but something wasn't right in her life story or her ambitions. She grew more preoccupied and vague and eventually we both agreed it wasn't a happy place for her. A van from her church came and took her things away to an apartment in Hollywood. She had a job as a receptionist with a chiropractor and took, on Facebook, to referring to "her patients" and raving about how much she loved her family.

Lindsey belongs with the "Saints" because she did good, caring work while she could. She helped us through a difficult transition after the national church abandoned us and took away our agency nurses. She even colored Easter eggs with the grandchildren.

Mariana

Raymond introduced us to Mariana, the daughter of his good friend and a graduate of a four-year nursing program in the Philippines. She would have her green card in a couple of weeks and she wanted to work for us full-time.

She was a godsend. Competent and caring, she was willing to live in ten days and then take four days off to go "home" to a one-bedroom apartment she shared with her mother, with Raymond, and with various other relatives. The four days she was gone were interminable!

The green card never materialized. A scam artist had taken thousands of dollars from Mariana and her mother and produced nothing. By then her visa had expired and she had no recourse. She had originally planned to take her exams to get registered as a nurse in the US, but those plans disappeared into the same thin air.

Her mom had many ideas for how they could improve their lives and finally settled on a new husband who could secure citizenship for all her younger children, but not Mariana.

Mariana moved with us to our home in San Diego, letting me complete my last year of teaching. I could leave for 14 hours, trusting that Gary would be fine. She left to join her mother in a new scheme, setting up a board and care. The scheme fell through and, last I heard, Mariana was working for an agency in Los Angeles.

I tried several times to get her to join us for a weekend away or for a visit. She sounded eager and made plans but they never materialized. She said she loved us and loved the children. But her life was on a different, alien track. Her father was supposed to be building her a house in the Philippines with the money she sent from her work in the US. I only hope her future is brighter and more calm than her present seemed to be.

Colette

Colette was a very pretty, charming young woman from the neighborhood. She saw my ad for help in the workout room of our community center. She had always wanted to be a nurse and had slogged through six years at the local community college, laying the groundwork for a two-year nursing degree. (Cheap tuition and bad advising had been her undoing.)

She brought sunshine and good cheer, competence and a remarkable eagerness to learn to the job. She was great with the iPod and, with my blessing, set Gary up to watch "guy" TV. She managed the headphones, the eye care, the turning, the positioning with great sensitivity and grace and she talked to Gary, something that seemed really hard for many caregivers to do.

Colette's life seemed a bit ragged—her dog got hurt, her mom crashed her bike, her sister lost a pregnancy, her father's diabetes was out of control. She was seriously involved with a firefighter who had terrible digestive troubles and lived dangerously. But she finally made it into a nursing program and graduated with honors.

Martin
Martin was recommended by a friend who attended the same church. He was a brick—reliable, precise, caring. His main job was with an agency as a live-in caregiver for a very disabled, not very nice man. His wages came from the state and they were very generous. Martin helped in the mornings when his primary client was at adult day care. Martin admitted that it was hard to not be emotionally involved (the attitude recommended in training) with his "roommate," who had cancer, partial paralysis, and awful orthopedic troubles. Martin sold his Corvette (!) and returned to Kansas a couple of months after we no longer needed him. (His mom was there as well as a girl he really liked.)

Carla
Back in the Midwest, Carla was a licensed practical nurse (LPN). Her daughter is a Marine, married to a Marine. Carla came to California to take care of her granddaughter after her son-in-law was deployed. I found her on Care.com and suggested that she could bring the baby to our house and manage Gary's care while tending the little girl. This worked really well. Carla was super competent and more than capable of combining childcare and the care of my invalid husband. She caught medical issues the other caregivers failed to notice. She had the usual transportation difficulties, but I trusted her with my car when she had to

use it. It was pleasant to have the baby in the house and we got along well.

Troubles were forever massing on the horizon, however. Her son and his drug-addled girlfriend in Arizona had a baby who needed his grandma, too. Carla's second husband "back east" was fading from view and Carla was planning to transfer her credentials to California. In fact she moved back home.

Scare Tactics

I lived in a caregiving world of chronic, daunting disability and, sooner or later, of death. From within this world, nothing seemed sillier than the scare tactics of people hawking long-term care insurance. The urgent messages arrived weekly—you must buy long-term care insurance immediately or face financial ruin. This was a sick joke!

Or were the companies hawking these policies sadistic? Were they trying to make me feel like a failure for not having bought a policy years ago? We could never afford anything like the premiums the companies wanted, at least by the time we were perhaps prosperous enough even to consider such policies. We were committed to one another and knew that we would take care of one another. (The extreme of what that meant was completely beyond imagining!)

But the mailings insisted that within a few years a year's care would cost more than $100,000 and that almost everybody would need such care! Scary stories. It's like the news that each child you bring into the world will require half a million dollars in care. Cruel nonsense.

At the same time, AARP statistics, arriving in the same mail, indicated that median retirement savings are something like $2000 and that old people are mostly awfully poor.

In fact, no nursing home would ever have taken my husband. When he was hospitalized, he could not even be placed in a normal ward but was installed in either acute or intermediate care. Facilities for ventilator dependent patients are notorious warehouses for the dying and while I had my wits about me I would never consign my beloved husband to a "facility."

If we had had long-term care insurance it would indeed have paid for nursing support at home. But that would have meant agency support, which was unacceptable. That meant questionably-trained LVNs invading my home on agency terms. The supervision was dubious—see my Rogues' Gallery! They were often late, often dishonest and dirty; their loyalty is to the agency, not to you; they are often peculiar and difficult people.

In short, ads for long-term care plans (or retirement plans) and salespeople hawking such plans are not reasonable sources of information. Like the van sales and the wheelchair sales, they are programs designed to make a pretty penny for one or another company. Caveat emptor!

Each of us is on our own when it comes to giving care. Absent a welfare system designed to support people suffering from terrible, chronic conditions, it's a new frontier. You certainly can't go with the salesman's line. Remember that these are the same people who, in other mailings offer cheap life insurance policies with no medical exam for which my husband appeared, weirdly, to qualify.

More scary by far than the realities of our daily struggle is the huge industry built on fear that is allowed to exploit already frightened people.

Sub-Culture of the Afflicted

I didn't normally think of myself as belonging to a group of pathetic people. Perhaps this was foolishness and I should have gotten with the program. But when I would go there and lie back and let the wash of self-pity flow over me I would panic. I would myself become disabled then and stop being any use to anybody.

I knew there were support groups out there in hospitals and in cyberspace. But when I stopped by to check them out I felt so terribly sorry for all the people who were suffering so awfully! Especially the victims of abuse, caring for their disabled abusers, or for the parents of children whom they never got to know as healthy, bright, happy kids.

But support group or not, in the hospital or waiting in line at a lab, a caregiver like me gets drawn into the whole world, the whole sub-culture of people who are living with unspeakable challenges. I had nothing in common with them except that I also had extraordinary demands on my energy and my heart, demands to which the larger world was oblivious.

A man who helped me with Gary traveled to see his parents whenever work permitted. His father, who had advanced diabetes, had lost both legs and the surgery wasn't healing. His mom was struggling to care for her husband at home.

A kind and gentle pastor friend who visited us regularly was devastated by the violent and uncontrollable pain his wife—who was on dialysis—suffered.

Waiting for a blood draw I explained my life situation to the technician, an excuse for why I couldn't come back the next day. She told me how her parents had taken care of her quadriplegic brother for twenty years after his motorcycle accident.

On the elevator in the hospital late one night, on my way home after settling Gary for the night, a maintenance man told me he had visited his son in the hospital daily, for seven months. I asked if his son was OK. He said, "Yes, OK. Not the same, but OK," wrenching my heart in my poor tired chest.

The sister of a former student has devoted her life to the tender care of her daughter, born with awful cerebral palsy. She never heard her speak her first words or watched her take her first steps. Yet for more than 25 years she has managed her care and heard her cry in pain.

Every night we hear about the terrible injuries of the veterans and sometimes about the spouses and parents who are to tend them forever.

When a loved one is in a wheelchair, you suddenly notice all the handicapped license plates and the ramps and what is considered accessible at church, in hotels, on planes. On a more profound level you begin to suspect that most people's lives are touched by such affliction or will be before too long.

This awareness is not a comfort but more a shift in perspective, a new worldview. It's not the same thing as realizing one's mortality, that life is short. Most high school students seem to experience some such realization when they lose peers in high school—to suicide or car accidents or drugs. It's humbling, this solidarity with a vast number of people who give and give and give their time and energy to take care of those they love.

Support

Our adventure would never have worked without the financial support of relatives. Checks arrived in the mail in a steady stream—regularly and generously from my parents and from my sister and brother-in-law. Other supporters sent a thousand here, a thousand there, and one cousin and his wife contributed a really major sum. As the trustee of my mother-in-law's modest funds, I could apportion bits of money for bills.

I justified taking family contributions from relatives who lived far away by thinking how, in a less mobile society, my mother and father, my sister and her husband, would be able to spell me, to turn Gary and suction, to feed him and talk to him for several hours each week. Their money was in lieu of such physical help. I remain very grateful, of course. Their generosity kept the wolf from the door and assured me that I would not live out the rest of my days—after Gary—in poverty.

Not all families have the means to be so generous. I only hope that those families can provide physical support instead. Our daughters certainly gave us that, visiting whenever they could, taking over their father's care when they were in the house, providing fresh energy and faithful respite.

Sympathy

Sympathy in its truest sense is often non-invasive. It's a practical phone call or dropping by with a little offering. It's an errand or a card.

Perhaps it's reality TV or maybe group therapy, but there's some awful model out there of "spilling your guts" or "letting it all out" that is simply egregious.

The wrong sort of sympathy can be devastating. I recall, especially, the first months of our struggle, when each day came with fresh challenges, with raw new losses, with the dawning realization of what our life would be like in the weeks and months and years to come. Good, kind family and friends would ask in all sincerity, "and how are you doing?" or "how are you feeling?" or "how are you coping?"

To answer in all sincerity was to lose my composure, to fall apart, to burst into tears. This line of inquiry was all wrong, not at all helpful, inadvertently mean.

I didn't need amateur therapy, a time of tears and sharing! I needed to be recalled to who I was, really, to who Gary was, really. I needed distraction and support, most certainly not an opportunity to vent in some adolescent fashion. Hysteria was licking at the corners of the room; everything was about to burst into flames. I needed peace and strategy.

Acute, legitimate stress is not relieved by pounding on walls or otherwise expressing anger, despair, frustration. It is relieved by calm structure and reassurance that one is surrounded by love and concern. Even when you have no appetite, a bit of brie and crackers, a glass of good wine, perhaps a latte or a good piece of chocolate—these are tokens of care that are much more supportive than any invitation to bare your soul and share your fears.

Other efforts at sympathy are transparent efforts at obtaining comfort. Friends and coworkers who are truly grieved and devastated turn to family caregivers for support and reassurance. Sometimes I could supply this, modeling love and understanding, assurance and hope. Sometimes my resources would fail me and this neediness of the "sympathizers" felt more like leeching, like sucking my reserves of strength dry.

Eventually there are the roles—the excellent wife, the devoted spouse, the loving friend. These serve an important social purpose and we all draw on such models when we need them. I think we settle into the roles with a measure of awareness that they are constructions. So, as parents, we had idealized models, as lovers and professionals we held up ideal standards. To accept the role is to move from being the victim with whom others sympathize to being an exemplar. It stiffens your spine and serves an important moral end.

T

Taxes

For a couple of desperate years I pretty much ignored the IRS and the (California) Tax Franchise Board. They sent fierce-looking letters that I rubber banded together. Finally, I had to come clean and identified an amazing tax accountant with special credentials in clergy tax preparation. She guided me through the intricacies of both professional deductions and medical expenses. The refunds were large and more than paid for her help.

The hundreds and hundreds of items of medical expense all need documentation. Receipts, bills, checks, bank statements, insurance statements covering doctors, hospitals, tests, copayments, prescription meds, over-the-counter medications and medical supplies. All need to be collected, listed, totaled and put in the right form by the right deadline.

It's an unpleasant job. The sheer magnitude of detail is numbing. Worse, each receipt or cancelled check is a reminder of a person or a hope or an infection or a fear negotiated over the past year. It's the paper trail of disease and disability.

If you don't already know how to do so, learn to use excel or some other spreadsheet program. Get a friend or family member who's good with bookkeeping to give you tips. Try to stay on top of this awful job month by month or quarter by quarter. The result is money in the bank as your horrible medical expenses are all tax deductible.

Secondly, find yourself a really competent tax adviser. He or she will more than pay for the cost.

Third, learn all about payroll and state payroll taxes. If you have employees (as I hope you do), you must pay quarterly taxes if you're going to deduct their wages as medical expenses. My tax accountant handles the paperwork for a modest fee and then folds the payroll costs into my tax forms. (This is not necessary if you hire through an agency.)

Teaching

This was not a project I chose. Nursing was not a discipline for which I had any identifiable qualifications. My only training in home care was that short unit in the *Girl Scout Handbook* on the duties of a "Home Nurse."

I could, however, teach. Teaching was something I had done for more than 40 years. I could usually figure out how to explain anything to anyone. I could grasp the objectives and measure how well or poorly a student was getting the lesson. In order to teach, of course, one must know how to perform a task. I can advise and support a learner who wants to write an elegant paragraph. How to teach a caregiver to turn and position a very tall man, paralyzed and inert, with tubes in his neck, in his stomach, and in his bladder?

The teaching task was wildly complicated by the fact that most people looking for work as caregivers have had some training. They have gone through vocational educational programs where, I have gathered, everything is taught by rote. Everything is a procedure, done just so but with little interest in explaining why, little sense of purpose or common sense. It's like the miserable 5-paragaph essay taught in poor high schools around the US, or a particularly bad course in driver's training.

For example, there are protocols for positioning a patient and for regular turns. The goal is, evidently, a fetal position on his or her side, knees bent, arms both supported by pillows. Two hours later the patient is laid on his or her back. Two hours later the patient is turned to the other side. This is a hospital standard. It is not comfortable or humane but somebody set the standard and everybody observes it unless badgered and beaten up by somebody like me.

- I wrote long memos and faxed them to the nurses' station.
- I enlisted compassionate and understanding doctors to support my cause.
- I wheedled and pleaded and wept to get through to individual nurses.
- After a couple of days, I always got my way.

My husband made it very clear when he could still communicate that he had to be turned from one side to the other every waking hour. Delays were excruciating. To convey his needs to nurses took major effort since what he wanted went against what they had been taught.

So it was with the administering of medications (gravity, not pushing), with feeding ("bolus," not pumping), eye care, bowel care, mouth care.

Tomorrow

"So do not worry about tomorrow, for tomorrow will bring worries of its own. Today's trouble is enough for today." **Matthew 6:34**

This is one of the hardest lessons to learn, to bear in mind and to explain. Planning for contingencies is so very fundamental to managing a world of care. Managing inventory to assure that the necessary supplies are in place for tomorrow, for next week, for the month—managing supplies takes fussing about "tomorrow." Managing staff to make sure that all the hours of the day are covered, substituting relievers for a nurse who's going out of town or a caregiver who has a final exam. Planning appointments and tests is all about tomorrow, next week, next month. Financial planning for this or that contingency is fundamental.

These are tasks, not worries or troubles. Each is, with a phone call or a quick supply count, solvable.

The worries, for me, were the anxieties about when the next bad thing would happen—the spike in blood pressure, the next infection. It used to be the worry about this or that loss of capacity—first he couldn't walk, then his hands lost their movement, then he lost the ability to breathe, then to speak, then even to open his eyes. To stay in the moment rather than grieving over what had not yet come to pass became a necessary discipline.

Fear is itself disabling, paralyzing,

So it is with growing mental incapacity. You know she will not recognize you one day. Don't worry about that now! So it is with death itself. We must not grieve about what isn't yet a present reality. To mourn prematurely is ungrateful and inappropriate and an unnecessary sadness.

Not to grieve is especially hard when all your friends and family are so sad and want to pity you for what they see coming. Set the bar high. Explain that you can only handle the trouble of today!

U

Uncertainty

Interesting bits of pop philosophy occasionally came my way and I paused to reflect. For instance, Daniel Gilbert contributed something to a *New York Times* blog called "Happy Days." The title: "What You Don't Know Makes You Nervous."

A psychology professor, Gilbert argues that we prefer to know the worst, rather than just to suspect it. When we get bad news we weep for a while, and then get busy making the best of it. We change our behavior, we change our attitudes. We raise our consciousness and lower our standards. We find our bootstraps and tug. But we can't come to terms with circumstances whose terms we don't yet know. An uncertain future leaves us stranded in an unhappy present with nothing to do but wait.

I decided I was myself an expert, having lived with the most radical imaginable uncertainty for many years. I decided this advice is bogus, falsely grounded in our perceived need for a perfectly unreasonable certainty. Nothing is certain! Life teaches us this. Weddings often end in divorce. Pregnancy often ends in miscarriage. You're hired—you're fired.

You save for retirement and lose the money in the crash. What you thought was a sure thing isn't at all. That's life. It's always been life.

In fact the drive for certainty is pushed by doctors, the drive to diagnose and to push false science. This push may provide a gratifying sense of control, but it's wrong. Acknowledging, in all humility, our utter lack of control is wiser and more certain.

Doctor shows on TV all resolve matters in an hour. Mysteries are solved. What's broken gets fixed. Sometimes the patient dies, but pretty quickly. Is that the model? Art models life? (I've read that the show CSI has affected juries and their expectation of scientific certainty. Perhaps half a century of doctor shows have similarly hyped our ideas of medicine.)

As a historian, I must observe that uncertainty has always been a central fact of the human condition. The randomness of disease and death, the miracles of recovery. She is personified as Fortuna with her turning wheel. Indeed, I know for certain that my uncertainty is much more the human norm than some fictional arc to a life that continues "naturally" and uninterrupted to its predictable conclusion.

Unkindness

I don't believe that those who are unkind are intentionally cruel. To go there is to despair and think badly of the entire human species. I must believe with Anne Frank in some basic goodness of the human heart. Or call it our capacity for love and mercy, an aspect of our creation in the image of divine love and mercy.

Nevertheless, unkindness is everywhere. Thoughtless self-absorption is the most understandable. So another person with a "handicapped" parking placard parks in a "van accessible" place. They aren't driving a van and their choice means I can't park to unload my husband in his chair, through the sliding side door, down the ramp. I cannot imagine that this failure is intentional. The resulting difficulty for me is just as bad as an intentional obstacle.

The raw vulnerability of the particular disabled person can only really be appreciated from inside. And every person is different; every stage of every condition is distinct. Still, it is worthwhile for any sensitive bystander—much more a caregiver—to try to sympathize. That means thinking through the challenges—in our case imagining the barriers and the corners and the access to outlets. Not to sympathize leads to unwitting cruelty.

Many times we waited for one elevator after another, waiting for an elevator with enough space left to hold my husband's huge chair with its ventilator projecting in the back, semi-reclined. I find it incredible that an able-bodied young person with a heart wouldn't get off and wait, clearing space for us. That never happened.

I never kept count of the many, many times that people charged ahead of us when I'd opened a door to maneuver the chair through. Or the number of times drivers cut us off when we were pedestrians.

There's an unkindness when it comes to design and even décor as well. A threshold in a doctor's office or a hotel room door could be a jolting, bone-rattling experience—just a half-inch elevation. Just so, that hotel bed built on a foundation meant I couldn't get the lift under the bed to lower my husband from his wheelchair onto the surface of the bed.

I sometimes suspected a more radical unkindness that doubted our whole enterprise, that thought it was wrong or stupid to support and sustain a paralyzed life. "Why doesn't she just let him go?" "What a nightmare! I would just want to pull the plug!" Nobody said this, of course, but the idea was out there in discussions of euthanasia, in opinion columns about end of life care, even in the hysteria about "death panels." Such an attitude insulates the bystander (or friend!) from compassion, dismissing the need for generosity and sympathy. (Of course I was happy to explain whenever anybody wanted to ask about our choices—explain that Gary was fully human, fully sentient, enjoying a life rich in love and pleasures, prayer and the NBA. To explain that he was not a dog or a horse who should be put down.)

An alternative explanation is that the effort of constructive sympathy is just too much for many people, mired in the difficulties of their own lives. They may be horrified or oblivious or morally incapacitated on some level. I was raised by a mother for whom walking was always difficult. The victim of childhood arthritis and its primitive management in the early

1920s, she accomplished a great deal in her long, rich life, despite constant pain and very limited mobility. My sister and I learned as children to fetch and carry, to save her steps, to anticipate needs. Our mother never waited on us. This had to be training for my later life as a caregiver.

My mother-in-law suffered from acute Alzheimer's for a number of years. She died after Gary had grown "locked in." We had a memorial service for her and of course brought Gary. Kind people have often asked if she knew about his paralysis. We have tried to explain that, given her very short memory, to tell her would have been to cause terrible sadness for a bit of time. Then to tell her again, devastating her again. To understand her disability and to be kind was to chat mildly and positively about the babies and her activities, not to beat her up over and over again with the catastrophic reality of her beloved son's life.

Some unkindness and neglect doubtless proceeded from the simple weakness of friends and associates who could not deal with the facts of disease and disability. They could not bear to visit. They could not look into the face of immobility and non-communication. When Gary could no longer smile but could still spell out words, he asked me, "Will people still like me when I can no longer smile?" I reassured him that, of course they would. Well, some people continued. Others fell away.

V

Viscereality

Viscera are vital organs, our "innards." What's visceral is also understood to be emotional rather than rational. "Viscereality" is my made-up word for the basic physicality of caring for another person's body.

On the simplest level, I'm talking about grossness, about ickiness. From infancy we are taught not to eat our mucus or play with our feces. We're told to wash our hands after using the toilet. Countless ads for toilet paper and disinfectants and sanitary supplies drill into our heads the disgusting nature of this fluid or that discharge. The AIDS crisis and its major euphemism "bodily fluids" further raised the anxiety level.

I am a pretty effete person, when it comes right down to it. It took me forever to be able to handle cutlets and chicken carcasses. Backpacking was fabulous except for the backpack and having to defecate into a little pit and then burying the product. I am really disgusted by boogers protruding from the sweet noses of my dear grandchildren.

Parents deal with poop and pee and barf and blood and general mess nonstop. But that's not the same as a grown person's excrement or a parent's diaper. New parents wade into the mess very gradually. And the baby is so sweet!

In a clean and polished porcelain world with indoor plumbing and plug-in air fresheners, we can live oblivious to bad smells or slime. Even sexual intercourse—with showers and perfumes and condoms—can be pretty unreal, hardly visceral. We can easily ignore the unpleasantness of the body and deny strong feelings of revulsion. Until illness intrudes.

Whether it happens suddenly or over time, bowel and bladder stop working as we expect them to. Digestion is problematic. Mucus is an issue. Nobody tells you what to do and a beloved body is really disgusting. These feelings need acknowledgment and as caregivers we need coping strategies.

Nobody much *likes* handling mucus and feces, urine or blood. Nobody *enjoys* changing foul linen or anointing broken skin.

In fact there is a deep human sense of the taboo nature of blood and bowel movements and the rest.

World religions have purification rituals especially bathing, to counter the pollutions of the body. Women are especially prone to impurity from monthly bleeding and the profound viscereality of childbirth. Women touch dead things—whether it's a chicken carcass or the bodies of the dead—so they especially require purification.

I don't know if nurses are aware of these taboos and these ritual requirements. I don't know if they respect the mystery of the body—

because that's the up side of this darkness. Perhaps they just tune out the unpleasantness and get on with the job. Home caregivers, however, need a handle, need some time.

When we left the house, I put the catheter bag in an old macramé tote. I don't think it's natural to show your urine to everybody with eyes to see.

When we went to church, I suctioned my husband's mouth carefully before getting out of the van. He could not swallow his own saliva, but "drooling" is associated with idiocy and overmedication; it's slimy and ugly and I tried to keep his drool a private matter.

When we had houseguests, I was very clear that they weren't to be around during the "bowel program," when I emptied my husband's bowels onto a disposable pad. Nobody needed to know the details.

Everyone must have his or her own line between the public and the private. Drawing it properly, usefully, for an individual caregiver or family takes reflection and practice.

In the hospital, when he was settled into a new room, the hospital protocol was to bar family members from the room for an hour or so. Then, when the patient had been transferred and was tidy and situated, the family was permitted to come into the room. This made me crazy, but I suspected that it came from the perception, however well or poorly thought through by the hospital staff, that they are the managers of the viscereality, the body in the bed, the bags and the tubes. Family is to be protected from all these gross and physical arrangements. This is, however, very untrue to the realities of home care. It may be simply out of date.

Because one of my daughters gave birth less than two weeks after her father was discharged from the hospital, I couldn't help reflecting on how, gradually, over the past thirty years, the viscereality of childbirth has been acknowledged in hospitals. Family is present. The mom is the main actor rather than the object upon which the doctor performs. The contractions and vomit and blood, the infant and the placenta are all a crazy visceral swirl. Dads regularly used to pass out. Now they cut the cord.
Care for an extreme invalid is as natural and as visceral, as normal and even elegant as care for a sweet little baby. Finding one's groove, learning

the practice, all the while touching, caressing the body, is as human and good as it gets.

Visits and Visitors

Several of our acquaintance planned to visit and simply never showed up. They had a good thought, a good idea, even an agenda: I will come and play the guitar for Gary! I will come and talk with him about local election results! I'll be by next week to read this article I think he'd like! But they never made it to the house.

At first I would tell Gary and we would look forward to the visit. My grandmother trained me well that surprises are usually not a good thing because half the pleasure of a treat lies in the anticipation. After the first few no-shows, I stopped reporting to Gary that so-and-so would be by with this-or-that plan. The disappointment was too strong.

I have probably been guilty of the good idea, unrealized, myself. Never again will I share the good idea with the proposed recipient of my kindness and fail to deliver.

It was hard for somebody like me to understand visitors. The first bitter breakthrough came the first year when I realized that one must never ever say a visit isn't convenient. Whether there's a medical procedure scheduled or a bath, whether you have plans to get out of the house or are simply exhausted, you must never say no.

The prospective visitor will likely ask if it's convenient, if it's a good time. Always say yes, of course, no problem. Any hesitation will be taken as a good excuse not to come at all.

Most visitors really don't want to come to visit. They know they should come but they don't want to. They are frightened and stressed. They have many excuses to offer themselves for not making the effort. A little cold might spread to the sick person. Another commitment is easier to keep. Surely that wonderful family is taking good care of the sick person and I'll just be in the way.

When you realize that the prospective visitor is really hesitant and when you learn that any obstacle or difficulty will excuse him or her from the visit, you must insist that the suggested time is just perfect.

It's a hard lesson to learn that most visitors are just performing an obligation. That you should accommodate them. That you should make coffee and provide cookies for them. That unless you want to be totally abandoned, you will nurture and comfort and welcome and feed them. It's counterintuitive but no less true.

Our most faithful visitors discovered that it could be a joy, an inspiration, a heartening experience to spend time with us. One friend said she always went away filled with hope and peace and love. Another said she always left feeling better about life. His daughters claimed it was really relaxing to "hang out with Dad"—immobile, speechless, lying there and loving them profoundly.

A friend told me that during the months his brother lay dying in a local hospital—and he visited every day, difficult as it was—another brother excused himself from coming to the hospital. It was "just too hard" to see the sick brother lying there. My friend was horrified. The difficulty goes with the job of human relationships. You visit the sick and the dying or you are not a moral person. Of course it's hard! Sickness and death are hard.

Because my husband could hear but not speak, and because many visitors had trouble speaking to somebody who could not respond, a visit meant I was there to keep up the other end of the conversation—positioning myself on the opposite side of his bed from the visitor. I got pretty good at that and assumed Gary enjoy being talked "over" (like a good meal).

Visits consume a great deal of time and energy. They are worth the investment and the rearranging of schedules. They keep the awful sense of isolation and abandonment at bay.

W

Winning the Lottery

Sometime early in our ordeal I read an article, some bit of popular psychology or a health piece in a newspaper, that asserted that joy and sorrow, cheerfulness and depression, are innate. They are largely unaffected by circumstance. So, when a depressive sort of person wins a fabulous amount of money, he or she may be euphoric for a couple of months, but then the dark cloud descends again. The circumstance of huge wealth brings only passing joy. Just so, the author claimed, a fundamentally cheerful person may be daunted by catastrophe—the example was a broken neck—but will, in a few months, return to basic good cheer.

I remembered the article because, whatever the science behind it, it contains a basic truth: Our moral compass, our natural level of endorphins, our skill at making lemonade from lemons or, I suppose, poisoning the lemonade with tears and bile, these personality qualities will determine our level of joy more than life's circumstances—horrible or wonderful, painful or joyful.

This is not a simple perception because I believe each of us contains both depressive tendencies and joyful, upbeat tendencies. One or the other may predominate one day or one hour or one month. But the balance will be restored if we are patient with ourselves.

X

Xanax

There's absolutely nothing wrong with turning to drugs for help with the really bad times. (It's an individual judgment, of course, as to what constitutes a really bad time.) My doctors prescribed Xanax. I took only half a tablet and only once every month or two. (The pills crumbled in the bottle before I used them all.) Usually just knowing the bottle was there, in my bag, relieved my anxiety. I could deep breathe through the rough time or distract myself with a taped Daily Show or (when I had coverage) a walk to the park.

I probably resisted medication more than was quite fair to myself.

I used generic Benadryl for a sleep aid. Unless there was a daughter or friend sleeping over, I wouldn't take real sleeping pills. If an alarm had sounded in the night and I had been drugged, I worried that I wouldn't have managed the situation appropriately and the result would have been brain damage or death.

Y

Yes we can!

My husband was the adventuresome one. I was always more likely to stay at home, reading or writing. We shared a sort of critical edginess, a pleasure in new perspectives, but I wouldn't call my own tendency adventuresome.

He guided me through our adventure in disability. His lifelong joy in the out-of-doors encouraged me to get him out into the sunlight whenever possible and despite the crazy complexity of charging batteries, dressing and transfers. It reminded me every time of the intricate planning that went into Gary's extended backpacking trips—the supplies, the need to anticipate potential disaster, the spirit of trying something extraordinary.

I don't think of myself as physically strong, but I learned to do amazing things with my muscles and bones, feats of body mechanics. If I were to have injured my back or broken a bone, the whole adventure would have come to a screeching halt, with paramedics and hospitalization and likely death.

All along, it was Gary's enthusiasm for the untried path, for new horizons, for making it to the peak, that heartened and encouraged me. Just as he had coaxed me up the trails in the Sierras, so he led me on this wild and ever-challenging trek of disability. Special equipment, foods and clothing, expertise and can-do energy are at least analogous.

It wasn't an adventure either of us would have chosen, but we proved we could do it without any bad tumbles or dreadful parasites from drinking water or bears crashing into our tent.

One six-hour power outage tested the system. The adjustable bed wouldn't work as it had no battery back-up. So, before the lights failed, I transferred Gary into the zero-gravity recliner in the living room (using the battery-powered lift). The ventilator and the suction machine both had good battery power. The recliner could tilt mechanically, shifting Gary's weight every hour much like a turn. His iPod supplied plenty of reading material. Gradually, the light failed and I found a flashlight and some candles. My laptop was out of power. If the battery and the back-up ran out on the vent, I could call 911 on my cell phone. I had all the contingencies covered. But we were fine. The lights came on at 9 pm or so and I wheeled Gary back to the bedroom. These are the adventures of wilderness campers.

Indeed, I had hoped to get Gary into the desert, which he loved. Probably not in a tent, although I admit that I have fantasized about that. Then there was my dream of an RV with a winch and the camping cot adapted as an adjustable bed. It never worked out.

Z

Zero-Sum Game

A zero-sum game is a term used in game theory to describe both real games, and situations of all kinds, usually between two players or participants, where the gain of one player is offset by the loss of another player, equaling the sum of zero. For instance, if you play a single game of chess with someone, one person will lose and one person will win. The win (+1) added to the loss (-1) equals zero. (WiseGeek.com)

In my years as a caregiver I sometimes drifted into a game mindset. Most miserably, I recall once referring to the communication system of spelling words as a game and hurting Gary's feelings. I felt terrible when I realized how he had understood what I had said as dismissive. After he lost the ability to spell, I felt even worse remembering the thought.

I have also thought of our life together as a game of pretend: I am pretending to be a (bad) nurse, a heroic wife, even a necrophiliac lover of an inert body. This was all a crazy game, a performance! It wasn't who we really were. Talking with students about vampires (the Twilight series) and their religious dimension, I mentioned that I had thought about vampires and tracheostomies. (It's about the horrible hole in the neck.) A couple of years in we attended a Halloween party and a child, fascinated by Gary's appearance—the chair, the whooshing vent, his immobility—asked if that was a costume.

But probably the most game-like dimension was the zero-sum idea. There were days or seasons of our life together when I was the awful loser. I had lost so much. I had played my life for keeps and married a man who was now death-in-life, unable to help me, to comfort me, to dance with me or even to kiss me. At the same time, I had to monitor him constantly, hire helpers, be ready in an instant to rush him to the hospital. My fingers were callused from the turns. My heart ached. Every other day I had to empty his bowels. What was "in it" for me? His life was everything—rich in reading and music, entertainment and love.

Other times, I felt richly loved and appreciated. I had chosen that life, at least chosen it over the unacceptable alternative institutionalization and abandonment of a beloved spouse. I had learned so much, cared so much, grown in humanity and compassion for the many members of our community of afflicted men and women and those who care for them. It was an adventure and Gary had directed our climb up this particular mountain. His last crazy project! He was the victim, not me. He lost everything. I gained a world of human understanding. I have known the kindness of friends and the devotion of family as I would never have known these things without this challenge.

Perhaps the idea of a zero-sum game is inappropriately competitive. But couples are always in competition on some level. Early on, facing the enterprise, Gary said to one of the daughters that he was mostly worried about me. His support and concern, however silent his lips and impassive his body, were at least as palpable as my own.

EPILOGUE

My beloved husband died on June 8, 2011, as I was nearing completion of a draft of this little book. He died at home. His pastor came to read the prayers. I turned off the ventilator and removed the trach tube from his poor throat. I took out the catheter. Two faithful caregivers bathed and dressed him.

After a lovely service, joyful and faithful and beautiful, we buried him in a coffin carved in walnut by Trappist monks. The children put roses on the coffin.

I was sad, but also freed from all the constraints and responsibilities of giving care. I wouldn't have wanted him to live another hour confined to that poor, stricken body.

The learning continued:

After the funeral I slipped and broke my ankle. I had surgery. I became the patient, first in the hospital, then dependent on family for care. So many recollections came flooding over me!

I remembered my mother's dependency and use of a walker, her hunger in my house when meals weren't served at times to which she was accustomed, her distress at being a burden.

I remembered, of course, the years of Gary's paralysis. I thought with new understanding how terrible they must have been and how doggedly I had insisted on putting the best construction on his situation. He MUST have grown comfortable, grown accustomed to his helplessness and built a space in his mind for retreat and solace. To imagine otherwise is to disrespect those years.

But five days into my own lameness I found I could not imagine. I could speak and move, type and hold the baby. My minimal constraint was so mild compared with either my mother's lifelong dependency or my beloved husband's terrible five years of total paralysis. Still, the freak fall and the short-term inability to walk gave me insight that I would otherwise have lacked.

I heard the baby crying and couldn't go to comfort her. The phone rang and I couldn't answer it.

I seem to recall a sermon Gary had preached, one of his last, about how the world isn't divided between the able-bodied and the disabled. Each of us will face disability at some point. The question is when. And how we will understand such disability. Or maybe that's my retake on a sermon I know he preached about prayers for healing and recovery. He said we will of course be healed by the Great Physician—now, immediately, in good time, or at the resurrection.

When I began this project I knew that it required a conclusion, an ending, to be complete. Of course I dreaded the natural and, likely inevitable, ending at the grave. As a writer and student of literature I knew the ending was required. The book could not go on forever. My great surprise came when I was promptly laid up with my own disability—affording me the time to draw the manuscript to a conclusion, to grieve my personal loss, and to learn in miniature how it feels to be helpless and dependent on the kindness of family and hired caregivers.

APPENDIX

Daily Care

Preparation: 7:30 am

1. Mix food in large tumbler OR 2-cup glass measuring cup:
   - 3 scoops of protein powder in 2/3 cup water;
   - one capsule acidophilus and one capsule cranberry extract—blend with hand blender;
   - one can of Nutren Pulmonary (in cupboard, stock in garage).

2. Prepare meds in 2 plastic medicine cups:
   - one med cup: 200 mg tablet of Amiodarone, crushed and mixed with capsule of Gabapentin—and a bit of water to dissolve;
   - second med cup: vitamin C, multivitamin, baby aspirin, crushed and mixed with water.

3. Empty suction canister and rinse; replace in suction machine and test to assure good vacuum.

4. Empty catheter bag (urine), using urinal in bathroom. Secure clamp or you'll wish you had.

5. Bring bowel bin from oak cabinet next to the bathroom, checking to make sure it's stocked with listed items.

6. Turn on some nice music, using TV remote (941 is one option).

Wake Up Call: 8:00 am

1. Remove foot chair (supporting feet), booties (holding feet at 90 degrees), hip pillows (relieving pressure on base of spine).

2. Suction mouth—and trachea if the pressure is up.

3. Begin breathing treatment (nebulizer goes in position of green HME; breathing med is in white/clear plastic ampule stored in basket with pink sterile saline). Treatment takes about 20 minutes.

4. [Bowel program day only: Use trapeze and Molift to raise Gary's lower body off the bed. Put a blue disposable pad under his hips and a suppository in his rectum. Lower him and remove trapeze.]

5. Turn Gary to side—normal turn, 2 pillows behind his back, one between his legs—raise his upper body, release his shoulder and straighten fingers. Give him headphones so he can hear the nice music.

6. Give meds and food with a good flush of water. (Gravity best, use plunger only if there's resistance.)

7. Start up iPod playlist and make certain the volume is good.

Bowel Program (alternate days, at 9:00 am)

1. With help, position Gary on blue sling. Make sure he is exactly centered, with sling top positioned at chin-height, straps aligned, scrotum clear. Make sure the blue disposable pad is in position under his bottom (or you'll be sorry).

2. Loops: Use the blue loops closest to the sling for shoulders; use green loops for legs.

3. Lift with help: One person holds sling alongside ears to ease head into position AND to keep vent circuit in place. Second person watches hands and scrotum making sure hands aren't crushed and scrotum is clear of straps. LIFT!

4. Bowel may evacuate spontaneously. If not, with a gloved finger and a bit of Vaseline, move around inside of bowel to loosen

stool. Be patient. (I generally flush the initial stool into the toilet. It can also go in the garbage, well wrapped.)

5. After 5 minutes or so, introduce enema into rectum and slowly empty contents. Usually the enema releases a last bit of stool that can cause a mess if it doesn't come out.

6. Wipe well with baby wipes and discard all the mess.

7. Change bed linens—fitted sheet, draw sheet, fresh disposable pad.

8. Lower Gary carefully, centering him on the bed.

9. Release sling, move Molift, remove sling (either by turning Gary and tucking or by easing it up over his head).

Bath at 9:30 or 10:00 am

1. Gather supplies for the morning's bath and oral care: shampoo tray, 3 or 4 towels, 2 washcloths, oral care basket, new bedding, clean shirt, eye solutions, and an Aveeno cleaning pad.

2. Facial and oral care
Eyes—Flush eyes with saline, using one tube each. Apply ointment by lining the inside of each lower eyelid and massaging it in. Remove excess residue very gently.
Face—Lightly soak Aveeno cloth with water and scrub entire face EXCEPT eyes. Rinse well with a warm washcloth.

   Teeth—Apply a small amount of toothpaste to the electric toothbrush. Brush each tooth surface thoroughly. Rinse well, using a clean feeding syringe, suctioning water with yankauer (long, curved extension).

   Tongue—Soak gauze pad with water and leave on Gary's tongue for few minutes. Remove gauze and scrub tongue thoroughly with a tongue-sponge-on-a-stick. Tongue should be perfectly pink with no white residue.

Shave—No shaving cream necessary. Do make sure the shaver is clean and charged.

3. Shampoo
    - Stop iPod and remove.
    - Remove shirt, starting with one arm, then head. Pause to detach trach circuit and reattach. Then second arm. Don't force anything!
    - Position Gary so that he's lying flat. Gently ease shampoo tray under his head and shoulders. Put cotton balls in his ears to avoid fungal growth.
    - Wet hair with warm water and apply only a small quantity of shampoo and massage thoroughly. Rinse well.
    - Position towels under arms and legs and one, folded, under his neck.
    - Drain shampoo tray into reservoir and secure. REMOVE tray gradually, easing Gary's head onto towel. Dump the water.
    - Elevate Gary's head.
    - Towel dry Gary's hair, remove cotton balls from his ears, and replace iPod.

4. Tracheostomy care
    - Prepare a plastic medicine cup with half sterile saline, half hydrogen peroxide.
    - Set out a new inner cannula, a clean (trimmed) trach collar, a clean split gauze, two sterile gauze pads and two long, wooden swab sticks.
    - Remove dirty collar and dirty gauze.
    - Wrap swab stick in gauze and swab all around the tracheostomy site, including the tube. Repeat with second stick and second gauze.
    - Replace spit gauze, securing smoothly.
    - Attach fresh collar and fasten—neither too loose nor too tight—two fingers should bit between collar and neck.
    - Exchange inner cannula, moving quickly but precisely.

5. Bath
   No two caregivers have exactly the same technique. One uses a spray bottle, another two dishpans of water. Here are three principles:
   - Wash seriously. Real scrubbing is good for the skin and feels wonderful—especially the back and shoulders. When he could communicate, Gary complained about nurses who were into "dabbing" rather than washing.
   - Rinse seriously. Soap residue is a disaster and causes awful rashes that must itch like sin.
   - Moisturize with lotion, massaging it well into Gary's skin.

6. Wound and stoma care
   - Clean carefully, using gauze and the saline-peroxide solution, around the suprapubic stoma and the GI tube stoma.
   - Tape sterile gauze around the dry sites.
   - Spray bedsore area with wound care spray.
   - Dry with little fan. Pat barrier cream over raw area.
   - Sprinkle surrounding area with nystatin powder.

7. Dress in fresh shirt and shorts.

8. Reposition carefully to turn standard:
   - On side, with two pillows behind upper back, single pillow between knees, shaped pillow under head.
   - Raise head of the bed, then make sure underneath shoulder is "released," fingers of raised arm on hip.
   - All fingers flat.

9. Clean-up
   - Spray any stains on linens or shirt with "Shout" and place in washer.
   - Empty trash. Restock bins with supplies for tomorrow.

10. Snack
    At 11 am or after bath, mix 2/3 cup of prune juice with 2 tablespoons of flax seed oil. Administer through GI tube and flush with a good cup of water.

Mechanical Support:

USE TRAPEZE and LIFT to raise Gary in the bed as needed—after bath, afternoon, evening & bedtime is pretty standard.

Evening Care

7:00 pm—Listen to PBS News Hour on Channel 711.
- Put artificial tears ointment in his eyes, inside lower eyelid, to prepare for watching TV.
- Set up to watch TV—basketball or crime show or baseball. (Goal is 3 hours of eye work per day—headband, glasses, head angled just so.)
- Rest his eyes during most commercials.

9:00 pm—Dinner (can with water, 3 scoops of protein AND 2 capsules—cranberry and acidophilus—same as breakfast).

Medications: HALF an Amiodarone tab, crushed and combined with Gabapentin, dissolved in water.

9:30 pm—Administer third breathing treatment of the day.

10:00 pm—Last turn.

10:30 pm—Bedtime.
Goal of positioning is perfect "floating" at "zero gravity" in bed.
- Position really carefully, top of head at top of bed, all sheets smooth under Gary.
- Place hip pillows (those dark floral chair cushions) under his hips, one on each side, lifting hips up slightly. They should go in (under hips) about six inches.
- Empty cath bag and position at the foot of the bed—making sure the catheter is clear, not pressing against Gary's skin.
- Raise head of the bed to a bit less than feeding angle.
- Place small or thin pillows under hands for perfect extension
- Place one fluffy pillow under each leg, between knee and heel.
- Place feet in blue plaid booties, fastening loosely. (Tag goes along axis of foot.)

- Place foot chair against foot of bed. Place a pillow between foot chair and bootied feet so that feet are just supported, not jammed, against chair.
- Check alignment—that arms and shoulders, hips and legs are all as straight and as "released" as possible.
- Suction one more time if the pressure is up.
- Cover with a sheet and blanket—unless it's cold. Then use a comforter.
- Turn "massage" function on for upper body. Say goodnight and turn out the lights.

Normally Gary rests peacefully until wake-up at 8 am.
I normally check to see if he's especially cold or warm.
Sometimes he will need suctioning in the night.

www.ingramcontent.com/pod-product-compliance
Lightning Source LLC
Chambersburg PA
CBHW030854180526
45163CB00004B/1566